P9-BIZ-881

*Modern Technology and Information
Make it Possible for You to...*

SNORE

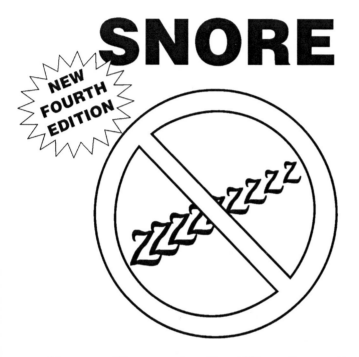

NEW
FOURTH
EDITION

NO MORE!™

*How to Help Your Family Members, Friends or Roommate
Stop Snoring and Live Longer, Healthier and Happier!*

JAMES L. MOSLEY

Foreword by R. Michael Alvarez, DDS, OSB, AADSM; Lawrence E. Kline, DO,
FACP, FCCP, D.ABSM; Kingsman P. Strohl, MD, D.ABSM

SNORE NO MORE!™

Fourth Edition

©Copyright 1990, 1997, 2006 by James L. Mosley

ISBN 978-1-884687-67-9

Copyright 2007 by James L. Mosley

Printed in the United States of America

All Rights Reserved. No part of this book (including text, interior design, cover design and illustrations) may be reproduced or transmitted in any form, by any means; (electronic, photocopying, recording, Internet, e-mail, or otherwise) without prior written permission of the publisher. No parts of this book may be translated into another language without the prior written permission of the publisher. Making copies of any part of this book for any purpose other than your personal use is a violation of the United States and International copyright laws.

International Scene Publishing Company

1220 Rosecrans Street

Suite 411

San Diego, CA 92106

www.snorenomore3.com

TABLE OF CONTENTS

Acknowledgments

First, I pay thanks to the Wonderful Counselor!
The number of people who have encouraged and
supported me in the preparation of this book have
been numerous. I thank them all, and am
especially grateful to the following:
my brother, William Mosley, for his artwork;
Abigail Amber Mosley;
Country Lane Graphics and Design;
Florence Biros;
Bernice Winn;
Gloria Clover;
The Respironics Sleep and Respiratory Research Foundation
(Sponsor)
and all those professionals concerned with sleep disorders
who contributed to this book.

Preface

This fourth edition of *Snore No More!* has been published through a process consistent with the author's belief in keeping current with new technologies, techniques, and treatments which are currently in use by researchers and health-care providers in the sleep disorders field.

Aside from providing information on the causes and treatments of snoring and a potentially life-threatening sleep disorder called obstructive sleep apnea (OSA), this edition includes a Snorer's First Line Responders (SFLR) Quiz, a Snoring Assessment Study, and a Sleep Questionnaire, which can be found in Chapter 5. The purpose of these sleep aids is to heighten the awareness of the snorer concerning how loud, erratic, frequent, or disruptive one's snoring may be. In addition, a glossary has been added to facilitate defining acronyms and medical terms used repeatedly in this book.

Empowerment of Family Members and Friends

After answering questions on many different radio and television call-in programs, the author has concluded that about 80% of the common questions concerning snoring and sleep apnea come from concerned mates, family members, friends, roommates, and coworkers of snorers. Therefore, the focus of this book has shifted slightly from its earlier editions to include the mate, family members, and friends in a more proactive role in helping to identify sleep apnea symptoms. By empowering them to be knowledgeable encouragers of sleep disorder testing, treatment, and compliance, their support of those afflicted with snoring and sleep apnea is essential and could mean the difference between life and death for a friend or loved one.

If the refrigerator in your home begins to make an unusual rumbling, every member of the family becomes concerned. If the noise becomes louder and more frequent, a service technician is promptly called to diagnose the appliance's problem. In the same fashion, if a person in the family makes a loud noise while sleeping, family members should react with even greater alarm. In a loving and caring way, combined with a sense of urgency, family members should encourage the snorer to seek medical attention and get the condition "repaired." This fourth edition strongly encourages individuals to manage aggressively their health and health care.

Dental Sleep Medicine

This edition introduces dental sleep medicine, which is a rapidly growing practice that uses non-invasive, reversible oral appliances to treat snoring and OSA. These appliances resemble athletic mouth-guards and are worn at night to treat snoring and OSA.

Increasing numbers of dentist throughout the USA, Canada, and the United Kingdom are trained in dental sleep medicine. The American Academy of Dental Sleep Medicine (AADSM) reported that approximately 40 oral appliances have been approved through the Food and Drug Administration (FDA) for treatment of snoring and/or sleep apnea.

Cutting-edge Technology

This edition also reveals the cutting-edge technology currently in use by doctors to screen, diagnose, and treat snoring and OSA.

The National Commission on Sleep Disorders Research has revealed that 40 million Americans are chronically ill with various sleep disorders. An additional 20 to 30 million people experience intermittent sleep-related problems. The Commission estimates that 95% of patients with sleep disorders remain undiagnosed.

The problems of snoring and OSA warrant further study, particularly for sufferers and their loved ones. This book shows those involved how to assess a sleep problem, and then where and how to get help.

Foreword

By a Dentist Specializing in Sleep Disordered Breathing

I have used *Snore No More!* as a patient education tool since the first edition. I provide a book to each patient on their first consultation visit. The book is user-friendly and reads easily.

The adventure the author personally describes helps people relate to the world of sleep disorders. Approximately one third of our lives are spent in a sleep world. The quality and quantity of our sleep is expressed in our daily living.

People who suffer from sleep disorders, often cause sleep problems for the friends and family who sleep near them. The disorder causes many daytime signs and symptoms (sleepy drivers, fatigue, poor attention in class, increased muscle pain with stress, tension, anxiety, and poor posture).

When I review the sleep study with each new patient, I use the glossary of terms in *Snore No More!* This is extremely helpful to patients needing to understand their unique diagnosis and treatment options.

R. Michael Alvarez, DDS,
Board Certified in Sleep Disordered Breathing by the American Academy of Dental Sleep Medicine and past president and founding member of the Academy [AADSM]
Certified in Oral Systemic Balance Therapeutic Systems

Foreword

By a Noted Sleep Disorders Specialist

I am delighted to introduce this important book. *Snore No More!* was a pioneer, first published in 1990 with a second edition in 1997, and a third edition in 2006, in promoting patient education. This approach is vitally important as the informed patient (and family) who participates in his/her care makes the best decisions (for them) and forces a physician like me to remain sharp and flexible to patient needs.

So what are the major challenges today? In my opinion these are prevention, access to care, and continued improvement in the delivery of treatments (behavioral, medical, surgical, and oral appliance therapy). At the present time the prevention measures appear to be similar to those used for heart disease, namely exercise, maintenance of ideal weight, and adequate sleep. Access to care is improving in regard to health insurance plans, but the number of potential Obstructive Sleep Apenia Hyponea Syndrome (OSAHS) patients is causing concern. In addition, the costs of diagnosis and treatment are high and for those without insurance, access is limited. This circumstance is not unique to sleep apnea. Finally, the site for diagnosis and treatment, so-called disease management, needs to change given the prevalence of the disease. Not all patients will need a trip to the sleep center, and in the future it may be that in a specialist developed care pathway, the primary care physician becomes empowered to decide who can be managed locally versus those who need referral for testing. This model of care is not uncommon for other common chronic diseases.

So what can a patient do? The patient can become more informed. Sources for information are available at several levels. Books like *Snore No More!* helps get the message out and fosters ideas, debate and improvement. The patient should become involved, as an advocate for the undiagnosed and for improved health. Also in 1990 the American Sleep Apnea Association (ASAA; www.sleepapnea.org) was organized and over the years has provided a patient-oriented awareness campaign. The ASAA and the more than 250 A.W.A.K.E. groups that the ASAA sponsors are proactive in providing sleep apnea patients and their families with support. The ASAA participates in discussions about federal and non-federal research and clinical priorities, as well as testifies on issues about sleep and sleep disorders from the patient's point of view. This voice in Washington or in your state capital needs to be heard, especially when public officials do not realize that OSAHS when treated reduces risk of sleepiness, car crashes, and health-care costs, so that a diagnosis is a sign of a winner rather than a stigma.

Kingman P. Strohl, MD, D. ABSM
Professor of Medicine and Anatomy
Director, Center for Sleep Disorders Research
Case Western Reserve University
Cleveland, Ohio

Foreword

By a Board-Certified Sleep Disorders Specialist
The sound created by throat tissue vibrating during breathing was once thought of as cute. Catching zzz's, we said, was a sign of a good night's sleep. That was until we realized it was a signal that air movement during breathing was impaired. Snoring can occur on breathing in or breathing out and is a signal of partial airflow limitation. Sometimes the disturbance is slight and sometimes very loud. It can be associated with long silent pauses or apneas. The person affected is often unaware. It is usually the bed partner who notices the problem.

The understanding of how sleep and breathing affect each other has improved in the past 30 years. We have learned the problem is common and a wide range of effective treatments are available. During this time we learned to test and treat this disturbance properly. Research and treatment strategies have been vastly improved. This all adds up to helping you.

Educating ourselves from as many good sources as possible is a duty we have as individuals responsible for our personal good health. This requires reading medical sources such as the National Institute of Health sleep Web site http://www.nhlbi.nih.gov/health/public/sleep/index.htm written by experts or individuals who have had to cope with the problem and have writing expertise such as James L. Mosley.

Spouses, family members, and those afflicted with snoring should complete the sleep quiz and questionnaire available to you in Chapter 5 of this book.

The findings of snoring may be important indicators of

sleep apnea. Knowing this and treating it correctly can be one of the most important health decisions you make.

The best first step is to identify a sleep specialist who listens to your problems and can do more than just order a sleep test or polysomnogram. The identification of the specific sleep problem is the most important step and your interaction with an expert can draw upon that skill and experience which guides you to a solution.

Many treatments are promoted, and some sound simple and appealing. Yet, many simple solutions are ineffective and may actually be harmful. So, how do you know what to do? The answer is to be well-informed and use multiple sources. This patient-written book has a personal perspective not found in textbooks or journal articles. It gives you the experience of the writer as you look at snoring through his eyes.

Lawrence E. Kline, DO, FACP, FCCP, D. ABSM
Director, Scripps Clinic Sleep Center
Senior Consultant
Division of Chest and Critical Care Medicine
La Jolla, California

Foreword

By a Sleep Apnea Patient

Author James Mosley's book *Snore No More!* will open your eyes to the life-threatening conditions faced by millions of people worldwide who suffer from snoring and its related complications. This book was the catalyst for saving my life. I read the first edition of *Snore No More!* back in 1990. At the time, I was a very loud snorer and felt tired and sleepy most of the time. The information I learned from *Snore No More!* enabled me to ask the right questions of my family doctor. The medical care I needed was available to me because I was informed enough to seek it out.

I was blessed with a doctor who had a thorough knowledge of ongoing research in the sleep disorders field, and he knew about the treatments that were being prescribed for sleep disorder patients.

I wanted to be tested at a sleep disorders center, mainly because I had read in *Snore No More!* that loud erratic snorers who suffered with excessive daytime sleepiness should be tested at an accredited sleep disorders center.

I was tested and diagnosed with severe obstructive sleep apnea, which probably started when I was a teenager, because that's when my loud snoring began.

I now use a Continuous Positive Airway Pressure system that effectively stops my snoring and the excessive daytime sleepiness. I am no longer tired during the day and I feel great!

Snore No More! helped me to understand the steps I should take to get help. It also helped me to better understand the connection between sleep problems and other physical ailments, such as high blood pressure and heart disease.

Snore No More! is a must-read for anyone who wants to feel better, live longer, and be healthier.

Michael D. Miller
Maple Heights, OH 44137

Foreword

By a Sleep Apnea Patient

Before author James Mosley and his family moved from Cleveland to California, I obtained a copy of his book. I knew of him and about his book *Snore No More!* in a casual way, but I didn't pay much attention to it. Unfortunately, I'd simply placed it on a library shelf and forgotten it. The first sign that I was a victim of sleep apnea should have begun creeping into my consciousness when I would awaken some mornings to find my wife asleep in another bedroom. She'd explain, "You snore too loud!" But I didn't believe her.

I've always been a busy person, and as time went on, other indicators sounded warning bells that went unheard by my deaf ears. For example, I'd suddenly awaken nights drenched in sweat although the room temperature was cool. The next day I would feel sluggish, sleepy, and out-of-sorts. Well, as my maternal grandmother had always warned, "A hard head makes a soft behind!" So I admit having been a hard head about sleep apnea until January 6, 1996.

That day I'd had lunch with some heavy-hitting political people and when it ended I made a preemptive men's restroom stop and noticed some stiffness in my right leg. But I thought it must have been caused by sitting in a cramped restaurant booth through the extended lunch hour. As I trudged toward the parking lot, however, my right foot, leg, arm, chest, and face got stiffer and stiffer as the effects of a hemorrhagic stroke grabbed all those muscles and tenaciously took hold. The grim truth is I suffered a massive brain bleeding cerebral vascular accident.

Upon release from the hospital I quietly read *Snore No More!* again. I paid strict attention that time, and every time since that I've needed to refer to it. Jim later steered me to the Cleveland Clinic Sleep Disorder Center, and I currently use a Continuous Positive Airway Pressure system that helps me with my snoring. I still call him for advice from time to time, and believe me—when Jim takes time to talk to me now—I listen! I strongly urge the mate and family members (of a person who snores) to complete the Snorer's First Line Responder's quiz. I urge every untreated person who snores to complete the Sleep Questionnaire and Snoring Assessment Study immediately.

Leodis Harris, Esquire
Gates Mills, Ohio
Former Cuyahoga County
Judge of Juvenile Court

Introduction

Upon my first phone call in a search for a publisher for my book, I was not surprised when the publisher with whom I spoke burst into laughter at the mention of the book's proposed title, *Snore No More!* After briefly indulging her response, I asked her if she found the title of the book humorous. She answered, "Yes. Just hearing you say that was very, very funny."

This dialogue gave me an opportunity to explain that most people view snoring in a humorous way. Their perception is that snoring is something to laugh about, to mock, and to be a subject for jokes. But snoring can be hazardous to your health! It is often an alarm that signals some dysfunction in an individual's breathing. The effects of heavy snoring can be very serious. It can, and sometimes does, kill the person afflicted.

Over the years, I have faced untold embarrassment and endured much ridicule from family members and friends because of my heavy snoring. While in the Army, I was confronted on several occasions by hostile soldiers who took offense at my loud nocturnal noises. I also remember a time when I was a younger man and the humiliating end of an otherwise pleasant evening with my favorite flame. After returning to her place for a night of anticipated pleasure, I awoke, alone and abandoned. She had chosen to sleep on the couch to escape the noise.

The struggle to stay awake after lunch or during meetings at the office, the dread of uncontrollable drowsiness while driving home from work on a busy freeway, and the loneliness and humiliation of being locked in a "snoring closet" (self-imposed confinement in one's own bedroom) are all painfully familiar to me. Self-confinement is a way of life for most loud snorers, since it eliminates family members' sleepless nights and resentfulness. This exile also shields the snorer from becoming the object of ridicule.

Because of my heavy snoring, I wouldn't dare entertain thoughts of going on cruises or overnight camping trips, nor would I take on a business or pleasure trip that required sharing rooms with teammates or coworkers.

I am still very self-conscious of what I call the snorer's eleventh commandment, *"Thou shalt not snooze in public places."* Sometimes upon visiting a doctor's or dentist's office, I would witness a patient peacefully catnapping. I could never permit myself the luxury of a doze in such a public place. I avoided long bus rides and always experienced a tremendous struggle to stay awake on air flights.

Studies at two different sleep laboratories diagnosed me as an extremely heavy snorer with mild Obstructive Sleep Apnea (OSA). Through traveling the medical route of examinations and consultations for my problem, I eventually found a non-surgical method to silence my snoring.

In writing this book, my aim of *Snore No More!* is sixfold. The first is to send an awareness message to mates, family members, and snorers: **Snoring is abnormal and can be hazardous to your health!**

Second, I exhort family members and friends to get involved in a meaningful way to help the person who snores to identify any symptoms associated with sleep apnea. This book also encourages those involved to conduct self-tests and identify symptoms associated with heavy snoring and OSA.

Another goal of *Snore No More!* is to strongly recommend medical attention for individuals who suffer from excessive daytime sleepiness (EDS) and other related symptoms of OSA. I appeal to all physicians and dentists to include in all initial patient medical screening a sleep-related questionnaire in an effort to identify a patient's possible symptoms of OSA. Another of my objectives is to encourage the transportation industry, especially trucking, busing, airlines, and trains, to implement sleep deprivation and sleep apnea awareness programs designed to lead to the prevention or diagnosis and treatment of sleep disorders.

Finally, this book provides information on where to seek necessary medical attention and lists the most current methods used to cure snoring and treat OSA, including surgical procedures and non-surgical methods and products which I personally use and endorse.

This book is prepared from a patient's point of view. I have had over four decades of personal experience in heavy snoring and have researched the subject since 1979. In this research I have discovered invaluable information about snoring and its pitfalls and cures. Most information regarding snoring and OSA, however, has been prepared by medical professionals and generally is kept for use by those in the medical field. Such material has not been readily accessible to the general public, being filed in medical school libraries and written in medical terminology not easily understood by those not in the medical professions.

However, the results of sleep disorder studies are released occasionally to the media. Some medical facilities publish journals or periodicals containing information regarding sleep disorders for distribution to patients.

The Internet is a source for information, but health-related Web sites tend to specialize in certain disorders. Thus the link between patient awareness and where to get help is sometimes missing on the Internet. *Snore No More!*, written by a sleep apnea patient, is an informative, patient-oriented (easy-to-read) health-care book on the pitfalls and dangers of loud erratic snoring and OSA, sleep treatments, and where to get help.

Snore No More! is my way of coming out of the snorer's closet—and to encourage others to come out, too—to stop snoring and live longer, healthier and happier. This book is intended to be a general source of information rather than a substitute for sound medical advice or treatment. *The information in this book should not be used for self-diagnosis and treatment apart from a physician's intervention.*

Chapter 1

THE DARKER SIDE OF SNORING

The *Guinness Book of World Records* office in London reported that the current world record for the loudest snorer is still held by Kare Wakert of Sweden, who recorded peak snoring levels of 93 decibels (dB) on May 24, 1993.

The noise level from a still night in the country or a soundproof room will generate a very faint sound and a rating of about 10.0 dB. A "deafening" noise level in the 100 dB range can be produced by thunder, gunfire, pneumatic drills, steam whistles, or large machine shops. When the sound level of snoring produces a rating of 93 dB, it's considered a "very loud" noise.

Dick Barnett (not his real name) snores...loudly. As a result of the symptoms associated with his snoring problems and his excessive daytime sleepiness, Dick had been fired from 18 jobs in 20 years. At the time I met Dick at the Veteran's Administration Hospital's sleep laboratory, he and his wife were sleeping in separate beds. His sex life was almost ruined, and his family was mentally and emotionally torn apart.

Dick was at the hospital for evaluation regarding his snoring problem; I was there to conduct an interview for my book with Dick's physician, Dr. Barbara Gothe, staff physician in the pulmonary division at the Veteran's Administration Hospital in Cleveland, Ohio.

While waiting to see the doctor, Dick and I had a chance to trade anecdotes that resulted from our mutual malady. I asked Dick if he would share some of his experiences with the readers of *Snore No More!* He gladly consented.

Dick, a 5'6" tall, 40-year-old family man, weighs approximately 196 pounds. He has been married 18 years to his wife, Susan, with whom he's had two sons. A positive thinker, Dick is intelligent and well-informed concerning his snoring affliction.

He credits his wife with prompting him to seek help for his debilitating problem. "For years Susan suffered unbearable restless nights listening to my snoring, and was just fed up," Dick said. "My snoring was so loud, I would awaken my boys in the next room. Although they were only three and five years old at the time, they showed signs that they, too, were adversely affected by my snoring. Their problems manifested in frequent colds, insomnia, nervousness, temper tantrums, and allergies. My wife was having backaches, colds, headaches, bouts with insomnia, and a general feeling of tiredness. My marriage was on rocky ground;

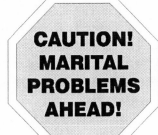

my family was being destroyed because of my loud snoring."

Tough Love Ultimatum—Get Help or Get Out!

One day Susan came across a newspaper article on "snorer's disease." The article detailed the story of a wife whose anger had built to a boiling point. She wanted to kill her husband because his loud snoring kept her awake. He snored so loudly, he would awaken himself many times during the night. His violent snorts and excessive body movements, along with his desperate gasps for breath, were just too much for her to endure any longer.

Susan, too, had come to a breaking point. She warned Dick that he had to be tested or get out.

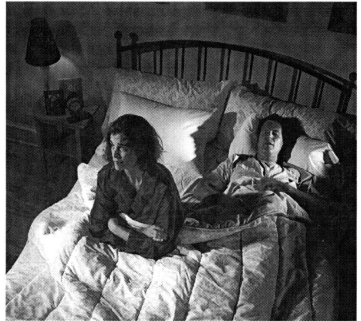

Photography provided by CNS, Inc. All rights reserved.

Passive Snorers

Throughout my discussions with hundreds of snorers, I have found that their spouses are generally the ones who encouraged them to seek medical advice. Family members who are subjected to loud snoring night after night are adversely affected, physically and mentally. They become "passive snorers." This is similar to the way a non-smoker is affected when he or she is constantly exposed to cigarette smoke. The following rule of thumb should be used by all passive snorers: Whenever snoring becomes disruptive to the snorer or family members, you should encourage the snorer to seek medical advice, especially if other household members notice that the snorer gasps for air and stops breathing for extended periods of time.

Family members of nocturnal noisemakers usually suffer symptoms similar to those of the snorer. They, along with the snorer, often experience excessive daytime sleepiness (EDS), lack of energy, and low resistance to disease. These symptoms can lead to other more serious ailments for everyone involved.

The good news that *Snore No More!* wants you to know is that there are self-help techniques that can reduce or stop primary or mild snoring. Also there are proven non-surgical and surgical treatments that can reduce, or even stop, loud erratic snoring.

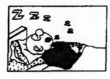
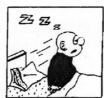

Overcoming Marital and Sexual Problems Caused by Snoring

Novelist Anthony Burgess once noted, "Laugh and the world laughs with you; snore and you sleep alone."

During our interview, Dick retraced in detail the darker side of his chronic snoring. Separate bedrooms was the only alternative Dick and his wife could come up with so that Susan would not suffer from Dick's snoring.

"Separate bedrooms were a way of life for my wife and me." Dick said he felt that his eventual move to a basement bedroom was the right thing to do. However, additional problems surfaced. He and Susan's already limited lovemaking became more inaccessible when he began to sleep in the basement and she slept upstairs. They set aside 10 p.m. each Friday as their time for trysts. From the beginning, however, timing was a big problem for them. Usually when Friday rolled around, either she didn't feel well and rejected him, or other circumstances common to most couples arose. Often he was too "dug under" to bother climbing the steps and would fall asleep before the appointed time.

Their ability to communicate in the most intimate way as husband and wife decreased and their marriage deteriorated. In spite of these adversities, Dick adjusted to his new bed in the basement where he had freedom to sleep without being concerned about waking his family. His rest was no longer interrupted by his wife shaking him when his snoring got too loud. This allowed him to get a full night's snoring. Consequently, he thought initially he was getting a lot more rest.

However, Dick was as tired and dug under in the morning as he'd been before he'd moved to the basement room. Feeling fatigued most of the time, he struggled to get through each workday at the hospital. Sometimes he actually fell asleep at the nurses' station during peak hours.

Dick candidly stated, "I just didn't get turned on as much sexually, mainly because I felt too tired most of the time. Men-

NOW THIS HAS GONE TOO FAR..... THEY'RE HARMONIZING!

tally, I would feel up to it, but more often than not, my tired body would win over my thoughts. Since my wife and I were already sleeping in separate bedrooms, this made matters even worse." The fallout from all this soon developed into full-blown marital problems.

Interviews with 100 habitually heavy snorers and their spouses revealed that 70 percent have experienced some sexual problems. Generally the snorer is too tired most of the time. Ninety percent of those interviewed who have snoring spouses indicated they had experienced some marital difficulties due to their mates' snoring.

Soon Dick began to experience physical and mental changes because of his loud snoring and its resultant lethargy. He was irritable, quick-tempered, and moody, which had an effect on his interpersonal relationships with others. His wife responded with resentment and rejection toward him. "She just didn't want to be bothered," Dick recalled. "In fact, at one point, she wanted out of the marriage, claiming I was becoming more difficult to live with every day. I must admit that there was much dissension between us, and my snoring was the main cause of the adversities in our relationship."

Limited Family Outings

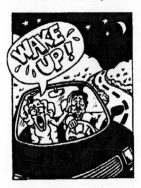

As for family activities, the family didn't travel or stay overnight in hotels. The one time they did go on a weekend trip, their stay at the hotel was not at all pleasant for Susan. His restlessness and loud snoring kept her awake until she finally retreated to a chair in the far corner of the hotel room. There she managed to get an hour or two of sleep. That was their last family overnight stay at a hotel.

Another reason why they didn't go on long distance trips was because Dick was so fatigued he would often fall asleep while driving. Susan would have to take the wheel. Because of the danger, Susan had to be constantly alert and couldn't relax while Dick was driving.

Dick's experiences parallel those of most heavy snorers I have interviewed. The use of separate beds is not the exception, but the rule. The actual statistics on separations and divorces caused by nocturnal noisemakers is not documented, but snoring is generally thought to be a hidden cause of many breakups.

Economic Dilemmas Caused by Snoring

When Dick said that he had been fired from 18 jobs in 20 years, he blamed snoring as the main cause. He indicated that he had worked hard and had sacrificed much to get through college and nurse's training. He was armed with the prerequisites for being an outstanding registered nurse, mainly because he enjoyed working with and caring for people. His objective was to be good at his profession. His ultimate goal was to get a supervising position to provide additional money to be saved for his sons' education.

During Dick's first year working as a registered nurse, he learned a lot and time moved by swiftly. However, he began noticing that he would get very sleepy at work during the day. While he sat at the nurses' work station to write out patients' reports, his handwriting would trail off to non-readable squiggling. When this occurred he had actually fallen asleep.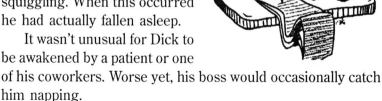

It wasn't unusual for Dick to be awakened by a patient or one of his coworkers. Worse yet, his boss would occasionally catch him napping.

"I knew that sleeping on the job was not acceptable, but I was helpless," Dick said. "I had no control over my state of inertness. I soon found out that the first thing my coworkers and supervisors thought when they caught me sleeping on the job was that I was on some kind of drugs.

"Some of them would make wisecracks or accusations, which implied I needed to get more sleep at night or stop whatever sinful things I was doing. Maybe I was addicted to TV.

"This was the beginning of a very difficult period in my

life. I had finished the long struggle of nursing school and had
married. Finally, I thought, the American Dream is coming
true for me. But my sleeping on the job created big problems
for me. My supervisors generally would issue me a stern
warning the first time I was caught sleeping. Thereafter, I
would be put on probation and, after several documented
occurrences of sleeping on the job, I would be fired. This
was very painful. Mentally, it was devastating."

Each of Dick's jobs lasted an average of one year, sometimes a year-and-a-half, before he was once again fired. After each job loss he generally took on another job at lesser
pay, which led to mushrooming financial problems. As the
money got tighter, his family's lifestyle drastically changed.
His self-esteem hit rock-bottom.

Dick went through some severe depressions, in which
he sometimes acted harshly against his wife, sons, and others.

Social Struggles Brought on by Snoring

As Dick shared some of his personal experiences with
me, we laughed about some and found others painfully em-
barrassing and humiliating. Because I also had experienced
some of the same things, it was easy for me to understand
and empathize with him as he talked openly about the social
struggles he had endured as a result of his snoring.

As an active Boy Scout leader, Dick had been his troop's
coordinator for outings. His responsibilities included planning
all sight-seeing tours, hikes, field and overnight trips. "Because of my snoring," Dick said, "I managed to arrange for
most of our outings to take place during the day. I took the
boys on beautiful daytime hikes through the woods and to
other events scheduled during daylight hours. However, there
were some mandatory overnight stays during which I usually
got severely ribbed and razzed by my fellow scout leaders."

"About four years ago, our scout troop was on a field trip

for two days and two nights in the middle of winter when the windchill factor was 30 degrees below zero. Some of us slept on cots and others slept on the floor. Five adults leaders and 26 boys were crammed into an area about the size of two rooms, with one fireplace that didn't provide much heat. The first night I was so cold I only slept about four hours. When I awoke the next morning, I heard comments like, 'Dick, your snoring rattled the windows last night.' Another leader told me that he had never heard anyone snore as loudly as I had. A number of the boys were whispering among themselves.

"I overheard one boy say that my snoring had kept him awake all night. One of the leaders stated bluntly, 'I stayed up all night, Dick. I couldn't get to sleep with all the racket you were making.' Another leader complained that he could not take another night of my snoring, and packed up and went home."

The next morning they prepared to leave the scout camp, only to remember that the scout leader who left because of Dick's snoring was the owner of one of the four vans that had carried everyone comfortably to the camp. They were now stuck with trying to cram 30 people into three vehicles. Dick felt responsible for everyone's discomfort, as well as concerned about how their scout administrator would respond to being short one leader. He also worried about what kinds of stories the scouts and the leaders would be sharing with their families about his snoring.

Dick arrived home safely, relieved to be back from an experience which, for him, was more bitter than sweet. Within a month Dick dropped out of the scouts. The ridicule and embarrassment he had endured was too humiliating to risk ever experiencing it again. Although he had been fulfilled by helping to develop boys into productive young men, his snoring had forced him to give up his post.

Thank God for a Devoted Wife

"My life has traveled over many peaks and through valleys," Dick said, "but because I have snorer's disease, I have experienced more valleys than I ever cared to. However, through all of my trials, my wife stayed with me, in spite of

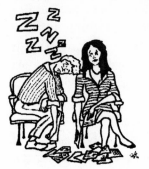 my loud snoring, my tired body, my loss of jobs, low salaries, and irritable ways. She felt like quitting many times. Looking back, I now know where she got her strength to endure the valleys.

"Susan is a Christian, active in church affairs. When she reached the end of her patience and declared she wanted a divorce, immediately she thought better of her statement and suggested that we seek marital counseling at the church. The spiritual counseling kept our marriage together.

"Susan's salary as a nurse came in handy when I was out of work or when my pay wasn't enough to cover the bills. Through all our trials, she didn't abandon our marriage. I thank God for a faithful wife who has stayed by my side. She has indeed been my helpmate!"

The State-of-the-Art Treatment That Put Dick's Life on Track

Upon undergoing a sleep study at a sleep disorders center, Dick was diagnosed with severe Obstructive Sleep Apnea (OSA), a life-threatening disorder. The method of treatment which he now uses to combat this disorder is a Continuous Positive Airway Pressure (CPAP) device, which will be explained in a later chapter of this book. Because he is sleeping better at night, Dick doesn't have daytime sleepiness anymore and is much more alert. His blood pressure has stabilized and his self-esteem is at an all-time high.

"I believe I am more pleasant and easier to get along

with," Dick said. "Susan often comments that I am much more congenial and pleasurable to live with since I started the CPAP treatment.

"I have moved back to our upstairs bedroom, sleeping with my wife the way it ought to be. We are thoroughly enjoying our reunion together. Both of us are getting the proper rest each night." Dick happily added that their marital intimacy has improved immensely. And, after all the years of disappointment and heartache in his career, Dick is overjoyed to announce that he has been on the same job for over two years and has been promoted to a supervisory position.

Dick's record of having been fired from so many jobs was by far the worst I had encountered of all the snorers I had interviewed, but poor performance and loss of jobs is commonplace among heavy snorers. This darker side of snoring is due wholly to the degree of the snorer's daytime sleepiness which is a major symptom of OSA. It is vital that the person submit to a sleep study for diagnosis.

Employers and Management Need Education Concerning OSA

Dick voiced a strong opinion that people do not view OSA and its dangerous symptoms with the seriousness they have for alcohol or drug dependency, epilepsy, asthma, or diabetes. He believes that employers need to become more knowledgeable concerning OSA and its symptoms. He indicated that the same procedures used to help employees with other disorders should be used to help those who suffer with OSA.

OSA Awareness: Webcasting Productions

As a direct response to Dick's concerns about management needs for OSA educational training, the author has developed a "*Snore No More!* Sleep Apnea Awareness Campaign" that will be presented via webcasting. These webcasts will link the host (the author) to organizations such as the

A.W.A.K.E. groups, municipal and county employees, management/non-management, unions, church groups, social groups, transportation, delivery, industry, and private company's employees.

Some of the *Snore No More!* Sleep Apnea Awareness productions will be live, with a segment for questions and answers. This service will be free to organizations and groups, and small groups are encouraged to participate. Visit www.snorenomore3.com for details and to request a presentation for your group.

Chapter 2

RIDICULE, HUMILIATION, AND PAIN: STORIES FROM SLEEP DISORDER PATIENTS

Can You Believe Snoring in the Bathtub?

My most recent snoring incident took place in my own bathroom. I was soaking in the tub, my body completely submerged, totally enjoying the soothing warm water. The spring-floral-scented bubbles and body rejuvenating solution put me in a state of complete relaxation and bliss. I had turned the hot water on, running it slowly to keep the water temperature as hot as I could. I remember soaking for about 15 minutes, meditating as the water invigorated my body and relaxed my mind.

I was awakened by my daughter's call. "Daddy! Daddy! You are asleep in there."

She was right. I had drifted off to sleep. "Yes," I responded, "but I'm okay."

By then the hot water had started to flow over the top of the bathtub, so I quickly shut it off.

She came closer to the door and said in a distressed voice, "You were snoring so loudly, we heard you in the other room. Are you in the tub?"

Before I could answer her, she shouted, "Get out of that bathtub right now! You could drown yourself, going to sleep in the tub!"

She didn't know it, but I was panicky, too. My mind was racing with thoughts. *What if I had been home alone? There could have been water everywhere from the overflowing tub. The slow-running hot water could have scalded me!* Other than a bit of embarrassment, I was okay, but truly thankful I was not home alone. This was one time I rejoiced that someone had heard my loud snoring.

On the Road Snoring

Some years ago before treatment, I was coaxed into attending a two-day church retreat. The men's sleeping quarters were similar to army barracks with bunk beds. Twenty-three or twenty-four of my dearly beloved church brethren slept in the unit. Lo and behold, the next morning the conversation centered on how much noise two other fellows and I had made snoring during the night. Because of the humiliation, I slept in my car the next night, which was very uncomfortable.

I also felt especially paranoid about snoring when staying overnight in hotels. If I were on a business trip with coworkers, I always managed to get a room on a different floor from the others. I turned the radio or TV volume up to muffle my snoring. One of the first things I always checked when I entered the hotel room was how much space there was under the door. I have actually stuffed rugs and bath towels under doors, hoping that my loud snoring couldn't escape the room.

I began to avoid activities that required overnight stays away from home. I became sensitive, to the point that I wouldn't share a room overnight with a non-family member. Camping trips and retreats were taboo for me. I refused to go.

Vicki's Story: Please Take Me Seriously

I am a fifty-seven-year-old female, and I have always had the loudest snore. However, other than snoring, I was an atypical obstructive sleep apnea patient (i.e. I'm not a middle-aged man with a big belly!) About seven years ago, I started falling asleep quickly and inappropriately. Watching TV after work one night, I awoke when a glass of milk

I was holding spilled in my lap. Sitting on the floor to clean my rabbit's cage, I slept for four hours. I could barely stay awake driving. I developed constant headaches. I told my primary care physician (PCP) that I had headaches and passed out. She gave me some medicine for the headaches and discounted my extreme fatigue by saying, "You mean that you are falling asleep quickly."

I felt as if a magnet were pulling me to lie down and I was powerless stop it regardless of where I was. I developed pain and swelling in my tendons so severe that walking was difficult. One day, I collapsed at church and my friends took me to an urgent care center where they said I had fibromyalgia. It was as if my body had started to shut down. My rheumatologist classed it as a rare arthritics.

Because of my depression, my psychiatrist called my PCP to express his concern about my sleep disorder. The PCP scheduled an appointment with a neurologist. I was told I couldn't get an appointment to see him for three months. When I asked if I could see him sooner, I was told, "No, because your problem is not life-threatening."

This was an extremely difficult time for me. My boss verbally abused me because I was sick. People thought less of me because I would fall asleep in meetings, but they never understood or accepted how hard I would fight to stay awake. I gained weight and my blood pressure rose.

When I finally saw the neurologist, he was unsympathetic. After I explained my four sets of chores, he told me I was doing too much. He did send me for an overnight reading using a pulse-oximeter, a device to measure the amount of oxygen in the brain. Ten days later I called for the results. The neurologist called me back because the results showed that I have a very severe obstructive sleep apnea. He had me tested that weekend in a sleep lab. Needless to say, I changed my primary care physician and found an excellent doctor whose specialty is sleep disorders.

After the first couple of nights with my CPAP, I distinctly felt that I wanted to go to sleep. Before I was diagnosed, I would fight to stay up at night, exhausted as I was. The technicians in the sleep lab told me that this is a common anxiety. Even though I was never aware of it, my body would undergo a life and death struggle to survive over 90 times an hour. It was as if someone were putting a pillow over my face each apneic episode. No wonder my subconscious didn't want me to sleep!

I have learned what the symptoms mean so that I can get proper treatment quickly. Further weight gain a couple of years ago caused a need for increased pressure, which I compensated for by opening my mouth during sleep. As expected, all of my apnea symptoms recurred. It took a sleep study to figure out what was happening, but now I have a full-faced mask and increased pressure.

I am actively losing weight and last year I started doing triathlons. I am a musician and attend frequent rehearsals, and perform in community theater. And, I have a new, rewarding day job. Obviously I am much, much better.

[Vicki's story provided courtesy of the American Sleep Apnea Association.]

Sterling's Story: A New Lease on Life

I suffered from high blood pressure and a blocked artery which was being treated with medication. For the most part, I got along well. About a year ago I began to feel tired and listless. I had trouble walking and doing my gardening. Then I noticed in the morning about an hour after I rose that I would feel tired. I couldn't concentrate on reading. I would see images. The situation grew worse. One evening I felt so tired I had trouble moving around. My wife suggested I call my doctor. They advised me to go to the emergency room. After several tests, the ER doctor thought I might have sleep apnea and sent the results of my visit to my family doctor who suggested I visit a sleep clinic. This was early May of 2005.

My visit to the sleep clinic showed I do have a severe case of sleep apnea. They encouraged me to come back and try a sleep mask. After trying the CPAP for one night, I went home the next day and I was able to walk around and do my gardening and yard work without much difficulty. I felt transformed overnight.

I have been using the sleep equipment every night without difficulty. I used to get up at least five times a night to use the bathroom. I no longer get up. I sleep the night through without waking. Now I have no more morning headaches or dry mouth.

To this day my energy level has improved a hundredfold. I do get a little tired mostly from trying to do too much, but that's to be expected. After all, I'm seventy-six years old.
Sterling Winn, Sr.
Canton, Ohio

Bob's Story: Downhill, a Day at a Time

I felt a little more tired than usual and I began to have trouble concentrating. My memory was a little off as well. No big deal. I had turned fifty so I could expect some slowing down, couldn't I?

At the same time, my wife began complaining that my snoring was becoming difficult to live with. Hey, how bad could it be? Everyone snores. Big deal. Then I began falling asleep in meetings. Not my fault. They should get some air circulation in those meeting rooms and get speakers who are interesting. I could find a reason or explanation for everything. The changes were so gradual that it was hard to see a pattern.

Some of it I attributed to my career. I was a Foreign Service Officer and traveled across multiple time zones. Jet lag was obviously one of my problems, and it was not unreasonable to accept that as I got older, I would need more time to recover. The problem was that I never seemed to recover, even after a couple of weeks. I found myself making errors in simple arithmetic, not following through on projects, and, in general, moving through life at half speed.

Psychologically, these problems and failures were beginning to get to me. I started questioning my abilities. Depressed, I isolated myself, professionally and socially. I didn't want to be seen as a has-been, or worse, a never-was. Retirement came as an enormous relief; I could get away before I was "found out."

Things went from bad to worse. No longer having a reason to get up, I didn't, lying in bed until noon or beyond. I dozed most of the day and dozed again after dinner. My snoring (I was told by all and sundry) was excruciatingly loud. I went to an ear-nose-and-throat specialist and was told that I had a deviated septum and my uvula needed trimming as there were flaps of skin hanging in my throat. Two major reasons for world-class snoring.

Dutifully, I underwent both operations. The second, the uvulopalatopharyngoplasty (UPPP) on my throat was horrendously painful for more than two weeks after the operation. I was now quiet, the snoring had stopped. Everyone was happy. Everyone but me. I still felt like a zombie.

I began group therapy to figure out the root causes of my depression and other mental problems. Over the next three years, I faithfully attended bimonthly meetings and also placed myself under the care of a psychiatrist who prescribed a series of anti-depressants and mood-altering drugs. I worsened.

My marriage deteriorated, and my wife and I began seeing a counselor. The counselor, rather intelligently, noted that I had been on a lot of drugs for a very long time and that there should have been some improvement in my overall mental condition. Accordingly, she referred me to a researcher at the National Institute of Mental Health (NIMH) to determine if a different "cocktail mix" of drugs might serve me better. The NIMH doctor took a full history (the first time any doctor had done this) and asked a lot of questions; he didn't just push pills. After about an hour, he told me to throw away all my medications and to have my primary care physician refer me to a sleep laboratory for a sleep study. In his opinion, I had a major sleep disorder.

I was incredulous. I pointed out that the only thing I still did well was sleep. I did it anywhere, at least 18 hours a day. He responded by saying that I only thought I was sleeping and that the results of the study might both surprise me and hold the key to my problems. He then commiserated with me and told me that while I did not have clinical depression, the condition everyone was treating me for, I was depressed, but with good medical reason.

The sleep laboratory was a strange experience. The technician wired me to 36 separate electrodes to monitor all my vital functions while I was asleep. This was extremely uncomfortable and I wondered how anyone could fall asleep wired up like "Frankenstein's monster." I needn't have worried. Even though it was only eight in the evening, I fell asleep the moment the light went off. At midnight, the technician woke me and put a mask over my nose (my first encounter with a CPAP machine to keep my airway open) and sent me back to sleep. At six in the morning, he woke me again and removed all the wires and other paraphernalia. Oddly, I felt better than I had in a long time. When I asked him how I had done, he responded with the usual, "The doctor will tell you after he interprets the data."

I prodded him for an off-the-record comment.

He asked me if I thought that I had awakened at any time during the night.

I said no, in fact I really felt rested.

He told me that during the first four hours, I had stopped breathing and awakened between forty and fifty times an hour with one peak of eighty-eight times! Unbelievable. How could I be so insensitive not to know that I was going up and down like a yo-yo?

Three days later, my doctor confirmed the diagnosis: moderate to severe Obstructive Sleep Apnea. I then learned that for a minimum of seven to ten years, because I stopped breathing during sleep so often, I had actually been sleeping less and less each night and had built up a sleep debt that was interfering with my cognitive abilities and affecting my emotional state. I was so sleep deprived, I couldn't think straight. He then told me that I had responded well to the CPAP and he would prescribe one for me. Having finally worked my way tortuously through the medical maze to an accurate diagnosis and the magic prescription, I thought my problems were over. I should only be so lucky.

My doctor gave me the names of two local medical supply houses and said either could fill the prescription for the CPAP for me. I went to the closer one in the expectation that tonight would be bliss. I encountered ignorance and indifference.

I presented my prescription to the clerk at the counter and he pulled out a machine and held up a template to my face to determine if I was a large, medium, or small. Having determined that I was a large, he pulled out a mask and said, "This will fit you. It is the standard mask for the CPAP."

That night in gleeful anticipation, I set up my machine, fit the mask on my face, turned out the lights, and hit the start button. Total disaster. The mask leaked air from everywhere. No matter how I adjusted the straps, nothing worked. Finally, I found one position where, if I lay perfectly still, the mask would stay in place. Unfortunately, by this time, the mask was so tight that I had an indentation from it in my forehead.

The moment I dozed, I moved. So did the mask. This battle went on all night. I was crushed. All that anticipation and somehow I could not get the standard mask to work for me.

Obviously I was doing something wrong and needed help, so I went back to the medical supply people. I told the clerk my problem, and he appeared to be sympathetic. He noted that the CPAP was, in fact, somewhat intrusive (an understatement) and that it took time to get used to it. I should keep at it.

His advice seemed reasonable and for the next six weeks I continued my battle with the machine. I did go back to the home health-care company several times during that period to see if there were other kinds of masks or if there could be some adjustment to mine. Each time I was assured that I had the right size mask and it was the standard. (Actually, this company, in order to hold down inventory costs, carried only one mask design in three sizes.)

In desperation, I turned to the Internet, eventually finding the American Sleep Apnea Association and the name of the A.W.A.K.E. coordinator for my area. He invited me over to his house and listened to my tale of woe with interest and a little amazement. He then told me that there were more than twenty different masks (now even more) and that one shape most certainly did not fit all. There was no "standard." After a lot of discussion and my review of literature, I decided to try a radically different form of mask, one that I thought would better meet my needs and fit my particular facial contours.

When I went back to the medical supply house to order it, they didn't want to fill the order as they "don't usually deal with (that) company." I was in no mood to suffer any longer because of their indifference, ignorance, and incompetence, so I insisted that they deal with that company. The clerk ordered the mask for me as I waited.

A week later, I was sleeping like a baby and my life began

returning to normal. I have been on the CPAP for almost five years and am so used to it now that it is as normal to me as brushing my teeth—and about as noteworthy. My memory has returned. My energy level is up. I have gone back to work on a part-time basis as an analyst. Life is good again. Despite the advance in years, I feel better than I did ten years ago. It's truly amazing what a good night's sleep can do and conversely what its lack can do.

A final point: You are responsible for your health and best interests, though it is difficult to take that responsibility when you have untreated sleep apnea. Some doctors have an understanding of sleep disorders, many more don't. Some medical supply houses have well-trained staff and carry wide inventories, but not all. If you have problems using CPAP, contact the ASAA as I did. Better yet, contact ASAA as soon as a diagnosis is suspected or made—before too much time, money, and effort is wasted. This is too important to ignore. Get the facts and make an informed decision.

[Bob's story provided courtesy of the American Sleep Apnea Association.]

George's Story: My 40-year Journey

I am a fifty-two-year-old male, married, and the father of a four-year-old child. I am currently a manager for a government agency and supervise nine employees, thanks to successful treatment of my sleep apnea. Life before treatment was not as good.

I was diagnosed with sleep apnea in 1993, the result of my spouse's complaints about my snoring, but it was not appropriately treated until four years later. Symptoms of my apnea included daytime sleep attacks and intense fatigue, depression, weight gain, memory problems, inability to concentrate, and more. Needless to say, untreated sleep apnea affected every aspect of my life.

As far back as high school and college, I remember I was always tired. Photos of me as a young child reveal dark circles under my eyes. I suffered from a deviated septum and engorged turbinates (the latter condition remains); both together nearly closed my right nasal passage and, I think, contributed to my breathing difficulties.

The problem of sleep apnea began in earnest late in 1972, during my second year of teaching public school. I have painful memories of repeated episodes at my desk struggling to stay awake. Yet, despite the undiagnosed apnea, I was asked to head a district-wide program on creative and performing arts and was appointed as one of four lead teachers to start a special school for gifted students. I even engaged in freelance services. My career prospects were bright.

Yet by 1975 my last year in teaching, I was constantly sleepy and I could not cope with the demands of the 450 students I saw weekly. Until this point I had been able to hide the problem from others, a problem I believed was of my own creation. Moreover, I thought no one else had this problem, no one could understand it—or even believe I had a problem, if I were to explain it. As my ability to cope diminished, personal setbacks mounted.

I resigned my teaching position in December of 1975 which created financial problems. Fortunately, family and friends helped. However, they could not help me with diminished self-esteem, depression, weight gain, lethargy, limited social interaction, poor decision-making on many levels, suicidal thoughts, and feelings of helplessness and failure. I was spiritually shutting down. The future looked bleak.

After leaving the teaching profession, I opened my own business, a franchise hundreds of miles from home—at that point, my only option for employment. I struggled with the vagaries of the new enterprise. I dragged myself out of bed to get myself to work each day. Photographs taken of me during this time painfully and clearly reveal the impact of my predicament.

As the problem grew in all its guises, I realized I had to concentrate on somehow healing myself. I embarked on a long course of ultimately unsuccessful therapy, and sadly, in the process of focusing on my own survival, I became unnecessarily estranged from family members who thought I no longer loved or needed them.

Pressures mounted and in the early 1980s, I closed my business after three years. Perhaps six months later I landed a decent job in the field that I should have been in all along. It was a major relief, and money was no longer an issue. I continued to persevere with my career and was even able to buy my first house.

Nonetheless, the apnea symptoms continued to worsen. I constantly fought sleep at the office, suffered from memory problems, and a growing inability to concentrate, and endured more frequent bouts of depression. My relationships with peers and supervisors were poor. For the next eleven years, however, through more successively responsible positions, I somehow managed to hide the problem of chronic fatigue and severe daytime somnolence.

My marriage did not fare as well. Married in 1985, we divorced three years later.

Fortunately, in 1989 I met my second wife, a trained social worker with supportive sensibilities and sensitivities to match. We married in 1992, and not too long after that, she began to complain about my snoring. My spouse also noted that I twitched and jerked a lot while sleeping, and that I seemed to stop breathing periodically (typical symptoms of sleep apnea).

Somewhere along the way, my constant complaints of sleepiness became attributed to the snoring. This was the beginning of the end of my sleep apnea. The first of four sleep studies was conducted in 1993, and my wife's observations of my twitching and jerking were corroborated. The doctor then prescribed medication for Parkinson's disease. The medications didn't do anything for me, so I did not take them for very long.

Soon after, I had a second and third sleep study, at my wife's insistence. They did not result in a prescription of any use, although I was finally diagnosed with sleep apnea. I suffered from more than 800 arousals (or momentary awakenings) in a single night.

During both of these sleep studies, the same well-meaning technician attempted to apply the CPAP mask. Unfortunately, because of my breathing problems and fear of suffocation, I could not tolerate the CPAP device at all.

Or so I thought.

After refusing CPAP, in hopes of finding another solution to sleep apnea, I made visits to pulmonary specialists and ENT (ear, nose, and throat) physicians, had a third and fourth operation on my nose, and underwent the UPPP surgical procedure (to remove my adenoids and tonsils and to shorten the uvula). None diminished the fatigue, improved my breathing, or even ended the snoring! The daytime sleepiness continued to worsen. My sleepiness from untreated sleep apnea was further complicated by my sleep deprivation after becoming the father of a newborn baby.

I again went to my primary care physician about my problem with sleep apnea. He recommended that I see another doctor at a different sleep center, which I did in mid-1996. Another sleep study ensued and I was again faced with the issue of tolerating the CPAP. Here I would like to make an important point. The manner in which the technician help me gradually become accustomed to wearing the CPAP mask was crucial to overcoming my resistance to it. Ultimately he set me on the road to recovery.

The technician did not give up when I said I could not tolerate the mask and air pressure. He employed a technique to address my complaint. He did not have me strap on the entire contraption with the air flowing full-blast in the beginning. Instead, with the air pressure set at the lowest level, and me seated upright, he had me hold the mask loosely against my face for just a couple of seconds. After several tries, I was able to increase the length of time until I was able to hold it in place for a minute or more. Next, while still sitting up, I strapped on the mask and continued to breathe with the CPAP device using the "ramping" feature. (This lets the air pressure start low before it gradually builds up to the prescribed setting.) I then lay down, turned off the lights for the rest of the night and went to sleep. While I did not awaken feeling rested (I think my sleep debt was too great), at my doctor's urging, I did purchase a CPAP machine for home use.

A month later I started a new job. Within eleven months, I was promoted to supervisor. Over the course of the first eighteen months, I received four cash awards, a certificate of recognition for outstanding service, and an outstanding performance evaluation. Above all, the best reward I've received since conquering sleep apnea was hearing my supervisor say, upon informing me of my promotion, "I wish I had three of you!"

The purple bags under my eyes are almost gone. I've joined a health club and now exercise more. My spouse no longer complains about my snoring.

For those out there who suffer chronic fatigue, snoring, and daytime somnolence no matter how much sleep they get, do not give up hope. See a sleep specialist. Undergo a sleep study. Persist in finding your solution. Do not give up. And if you have sleep apnea, by all means, give yourself every chance to get used to breathing and sleeping with a CPAP. It is truly life-changing.

[George's story provided courtesy of the American Sleep Apnea Association.]

Chapter 3

CONDITIONS THAT CAUSE SNORING

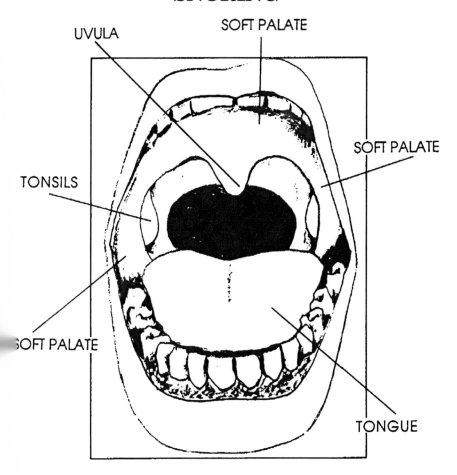

Flabby, soft tissues in the mouth can cause snoring!

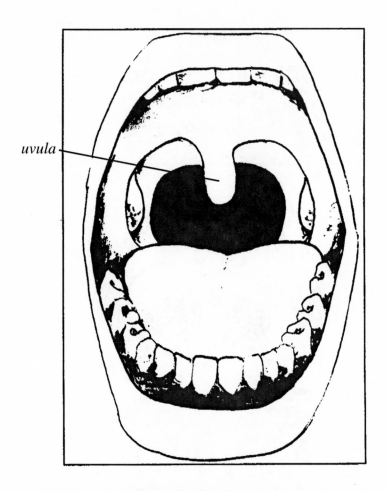

uvula

1. A long uvula may narrow the opening from the nose into the throat as it dangles in the airway. It acts as a flutter valve during relaxed breathing and contributes to the noise of snoring. An inflamed uvula usually caused from chronic snoring makes matters even worse.

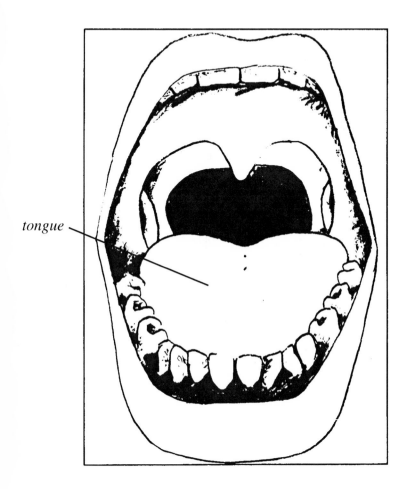

tongue

2. A large tongue can contribute to the obstruction of the air flow when it is in a relaxed state. The muscle of the tongue allows it to fall backwards into the airway.

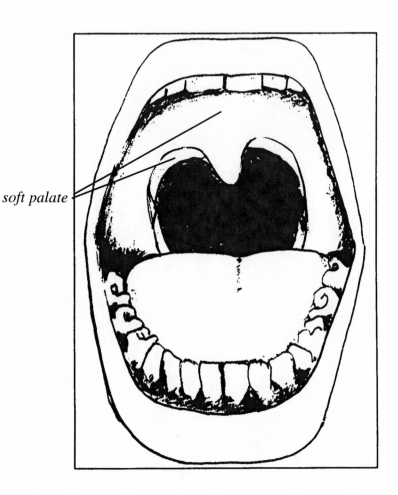

soft palate

3. A long, flabby, soft palate, when relaxed, could hinder efforts to breathe. When this occurs it causes the palate to vibrate and make noise.

large tonsils/adenoids

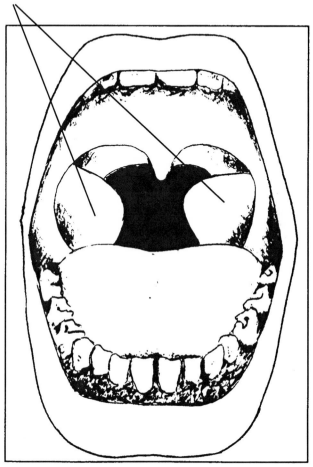

4. Excessive bulkiness of tissues in the throat, such as large tonsils and/or adenoids commonly cause snoring in children, Overweight persons who have bulky neck tissues have a high probability of airway obstruction which produces snoring.

What is Snoring?

Snoring is a breathing noise that occurs while someone is sleeping. It usually happens when the person is breathing in (inhaling) rather than breathing out (exhaling).

The source of the noise is a vibration of the tissues in the throat. The noise is produced typically by the soft palate, the uvula, or both vibrating against the back of the throat or the base of the tongue. This vibration is a rapid alternating opening and closing of the air passage which makes it more difficult to inhale. So snoring is clear evidence that the breathing passage is intermittently blocked.

Who Snores?

The results of a National Family Opinion Research Study of 13, 012 American households supports previous publications when it comes to the number of American adults who snore occasionally. The results of the study show that about 44% of American adults snore occasionally and 24% snore regularly. The total number of snoring incidents was about 78%.

This study is one of a few that considered both genders. There were no definitive reasons given to support the rise in the number of adults who snore regularly. However, some known factors that induce snoring are being overweight and the use of alcohol and tobacco. In addition, the baby boomers may impact the snoring incidences as large numbers of Americans approach fifty years of age. Snoring, sleep apnea, and other sleep disorders are more common as we age.

Snoring Incidence Levels in U.S. Population*

	Households with a snorer	Male head of household	Female head of household
Snores regularly	34%	27%	13%
Snores occasionally	44%	28%	27%
Total Snoring incidents	78%	55%	40%

Based on 1994 NFO research study of 13,012 households.

Do You Snore?

If so, you're not alone. Snoring occurs in all age groups, in both genders, and is heard all over the world. It's something you have in common with people everywhere.

Although snoring occurs in both genders, it is almost twice as common in men than women.

The likelihood of developing a snoring condition also increases with age. Approximately 30% of American males snore at age 30, and around 40% of all Americans snore by age 50.

Some people snore all night, every night, while others only snore when they first fall asleep or when they sleep on their backs. Some people only snore when they take certain medications, or when they have a cold. But no matter why someone snores ... or when ... someone else probably is going to be bothered by it.

Conditions That Can Lead to Snoring and OSA

Family History

Some studies have shown that a family history of snoring and OSA increases the risk two to four times.

Smoking and Alcohol

Use of tobacco and alcohol are labeled by researchers as contributors to the snorer's dilemma.

Abnormalities of the Upper Airway Structures

Abnormalities of the Upper Airway Structures include deformities of the nose and the nasal septum, which is the thin, flat cartilage and bone that separates the nostrils and the nose into its sides. These deformities are often due to an injury at some time in one's life.

A deviated septum is a condition in which the partition in the nose (the septum) is displaced so that it partly blocks one or both nasal passages. Deviation is usually caused by a broken nose, but may be congenital or occur for no obvious reason. Snoring is a prime symptom associated with this condition, as well as headaches, recurring nose bleeds, difficulty in breathing, mucus and recurrent sinusitis. If left untreated, this condition can be a major cause of snoring and OSA.

Individuals who have a facial skeletal abnormalities, such as a long face or a small lower jaw, have a greater tendency toward snoring and OSA. Also OSA is more difficult to treat when a patient has a facial skeletal abnormality.

Nasal Conditions

Virus infection, acute sinusitis, and chronic sinus infection produce nasal congestion. Virus infections generally result in common colds which can cause stuffy nose, swelling, and congestion of nasal tissues.

Some people develop nasal polyps (fleshy growths in the nose) from sinus infections, and the infection can spread down into the lower airway, resulting in chronic cough, bronchitis, and asthma. Polyps can also cause nasal blockage, making it hard to breathe. Most nasal polyp problems can be helped. While some polyps are a result of swelling from an infection or allergy, most of the time the cause for the nasal polyps is never known. When the nasal passageway is restricted during sleep, generally the individual will breathe through the mouth. And mouth breathing can cause snoring and OSA.

Allergy

Hay fever, grass fever, rose fever, and "summertime colds" are various names for allergic rhinitis. Allergy is an exaggerated inflammatory response to a foreign substance which, in the case of stuffy nose, is usually pollen, animal dander, mold or some element in house dust. Foods sometimes play a troublesome role. Pollen from trees and grasses or late summer weeds like ragweed cause problems. House dust and mold can cause nasal congestion. These conditions that make breathing more difficult can also cause snoring and OSA if left untreated.

Vasomotor Rhinitis

This condition affects the mucus membranes that line the

nose. The symptoms are runny nose, sneezing, and postnasal drip, which can cause blockage in one nostril passage or partial restriction of both nostrils. When nasal blockage or restriction occur, it can induce snoring and OSA.

Falls Asleep Fast

The speed in which an individual falls asleep also seems to correlate with snoring and OSA, namely falling asleep in fewer than five minutes.

Overweight and Obese

Being overweight or obese are risk factors for snoring and OSA. Snoring and OSA is more common in overweight people. However, not all snorers and sleep apnea patients are overweight.

A large neck circumference, usually associated with obesity, is a strong indicator of a potential snorer. For men, a 17-inch or greater neck circumference puts them at risk; for women, it is a 16-inch circumference. Large neck girth in both men and women snorers is highly predictive of sleep apnea. When the neck size gets larger, so do the tissues inside the mouth and throat airway. Enlarged tissues such as the soft palate, uvula, and tongue can cause serious obstructions in the throat airway, which can result in snoring and obstructive sleep apnea.

Obesity, particularly upper body obesity, is a risk factor for sleep apnea and has been shown to have a significant effect on its severity. Most sleep apnea patients are obese, when obesity is defined as greater than 120 percent of ideal body weight.

Can Chronic Snoring and Sleep Apnea Cause Overweight and Obesity Problems?

A recent study suggests that chronic sleep deprivation may be part of America's alarming overweight and obesity problems. The number one symptom associated with snoring/sleep apnea is excessive daytime sleepiness.

Researchers revealed that a lack of sleep or poor quality of sleep has a direct effect on the "appetite control" hormone leptin. Leptin is a neurotransitter produced by fat cells and is involved in the regulation of appetite. It is a widely studied hormone, thought to be the secret to overweight and obesity. Leptin levels tell the brain when the body does or doesn't need more food.

Research indicates that during periods of sleep deprivation, low leptin levels tell the brain there is a shortage of food, then there is an increase in appetite. Conversely, when leptin levels are higher, the brain is notified that the body is getting enough food. Research study suggests that during periods of sleep deprivation, the decrease in leptin levels cause an erroneous signal to the brain that more food is needed, when in fact enough food has been eaten. And this further suggests that during periods of sleep deprivation, we tend to over eat.

It is critical that people who are chronic snorers with sleep apnea symptoms should see their doctor or a board certified sleep specialist for a possible sleep study and treatment. Proper treatment should eliminate excessive daytime sleepiness and improve the person's overall health (including weight). Treatment will also help associated medical problems such as high blood pressure and reduce the risk for heart attack, stroke, and diabetes. The quality of sleep for the individual and for his/her entire family should improve as a result of the snorer's treatment.

Age and Gender Factor

The prevalence of snoring/OSA is greater in the older population, apparently peaking in 60-year-old men and women and declining in older individuals. Men also are more likely to develop sleep disordered breathing. It is estimated that nearly half of all males over 40 snore habitually. Researchers indicate that among adults, the ratio of male snorers versus female is 2 to 1. Snoring and OSA increases in women after age 50.

Women—Lifestyle and Menopause

Women are affected equally as men by (preventable) adverse lifestyles that can cause snoring and OSA, such as, overweight, obesity, and the use of tobacco and alcohol. As with men, a family history of sleep disordered breathing (SDB) increases the risk for women also.

Although research indicates that snoring is more common in men, once a women goes through menopause and loses the little-understood protection afforded by progesterone, the ratio gap for snoring and OSA between men and women appears to become even.

Because being overweight is a risk factor for snoring and OSA, the increase in abdominal fat during menopause may be one reason menopausal women are 3.5 times as likely to get this sleep disorder. Some attribute the prevalence to hormonal changes such as the decrease in progesterone. Studies have also found that OSA is associated with increased blood pressure, a risk for cardiovascular disease and stroke. If any of these symptoms appear, it is (life-threatening) important to address them with your doctor and/or a board certified sleep specialist. A number of effective treatment approaches are available, which are discussed in this book.

Race

Race also predisposes a person to being a sufferer of snoring and/or OSA. Studies show that African Americans, Mexican Americans, and Pacific Islanders have a greater prevalence of snoring/OSA than do Caucasians.

African Americans at Higher Risk

Data from a Cleveland, Ohio, family study suggests that young African-Americans may be at increased risk for sleep apnea. The case-control study of sleep disordered breathing (SDB) involved 225 African-Americans and 622 Caucasians, ages two to 86 years. They were studied with an overnight home sleep-study, questionnaires, and physical measurements (size). The results showed that African-Americans with SDB were younger than Caucasians with SDB (37 versus 46 years of age). In subjects under 25 years, the respiratory disturbance index (RDI) and the increased apneic activity (IAA) prevalence were higher in African-Americans.

This study supports an earlier medical review titled, "Recognition of Obstructive Sleep Apnea," published by Kingman P. Strohl, MD and Susan Redline, MD, MPH, which suggested that African-Americans could be a group at particularly high risk for obstructive sleep apnea, and the effects and complications related to their increased prevalence of hypertension and renal disease. The high risk of young African-Americans to sleep apnea may also be linked to alcohol exposure and/or tobacco use.

The review also points out that other populations in which a high prevalence of obstructive sleep apnea is suspected are Mexican-Americans and Pacific Islanders. In these populations, the attributing factors of obesity, hypertension, and non-insulin-dependent diabetes are more prevalent than in Caucasians.

Kingman P. Strohl, MD, is a Professor of Medicine and Susan Redline, MD, MPH, is an Associate Professor of Medicine at Case Western Reserve University School of Medicine, Cleveland Veterans Affairs Medical Center, Cleveland, Ohio.

Epidemic That Can Be Silenced

Excerpts from an article published by Dr. Daniel E. Cohen, titled, "Snoring, an Epidemic That Can Be Silenced" provides highlights about snoring:

A National Family Opinion poll revealed that 90 million Americans over the age of 18 snore, 37 million of them on a chronic basis. However, that same poll also showed that only four percent of Americans have sought treatment. Why do so many tolerate this racket in their bedroom? It's probably because most people believe snoring is simply a social nuisance.

Snoring Defined

Is snoring an illness? No, but it is a medical symptom, just as a cough can be a symptom of tuberculosis or the flu. Medical illnesses produce symptoms, and any given symptom may be due to a variety of illnesses.

Snoring is associated with a number of illnesses ranging from the common cold and allergies to sleep apnea. These illnesses all have one thing in common—they interfere with normal breathing during sleep.

When awake and upright, most people breathe through their noses (although mouth breathing is often necessary to draw in more air, particularly during exertion). When asleep, however, normal breathing is equated to nasal breathing; and air flows through the nose into the throat, which is in essence a muscular tube that is more relaxed during sleep.

Most people have sufficient space in the throat to allow air to flow easily. Unfortunately, there are several factors that, either alone or in combination, may cause the throat to collapse, reducing or eliminating air flow. They include anatomic abnormalities which constrict the air space, such as excess fat deposits, swollen tonsils, and other structural problems. Also, mouth breathing reduces the air space in the throat to the muscles in the back of the throat.

Most snoring takes place during mouth breathing.

Snoring noise occurs when tissues in the throat flap against each other as air passes between them into the trachea en route to the lungs. When airflow is blocked completely, an apnea (cessation of airflow) occurs. Therefore, apnea occurs when there is a complete closure of the throat, while snoring results from only a partial closure.

Because the throat is a collapsible muscular tube, a vacuum can form within the space. This vacuum normally occurs with each breath and exerts a pulling force on the tissues. The throat doesn't collapse with each breath, but making a greater effort to breathe increases the vacuum effect, which in turn can pull the throat closed, particularly if any structural problems of the throat coexist.

Surprisingly, even a stuffy nose associated with the common cold can create this type of problem. All the air that fills the lungs must pass through the nasal valve area at the back of each nostril. The nasal valve is only one-tenth of an inch wide and can be easily blocked by a cold, allergies, or a deviated nasal septum. In these situations, making the added effort to inhale increases the vacuum in the throat and may result in snoring and even apnea.

Normal Breathing and Primary Snoring

Upper Airway Resistance Syndrome (UARS) is controversial among some sleep specialists. It is apparent obstructed breathing without a decrease in arterial oxygen as measured by a pulse oximeter and is associated with frequent arousal from sleep. Some sleep specialists believe that UARS at some point becomes abnormal snoring.

Normal breathing must continue at all times, whether a person is awake or asleep. The act of breathing is an automatic, highly regulated mechanical function of the body. In healthy sleeping individuals, most muscle and neural activities will slow or even shut down, but respiration goes on under a neuromuscular "auto pilot." However, if something goes wrong with the auto pilot during sleep, breathing may become erratic and inefficient.

Abnormal Snoring
(Obstructive Sleep Hypopnea and Obstructive Sleep Apnea)

A sleep test must be conducted to determine if snoring is simple primary snoring or if it's abnormal snoring.

When snoring occurs for ten seconds or longer, it can cause a decrease in oxygen in the red blood cells, and typically frequent arousals from sleep. This more clinically serious type of snoring is called obstructive sleep hypopnea (OSH). OSH is usually associated with moderate to loud snoring sounds. Obstructive Sleep Apnea (OSA) is usually associated with quiet pauses in breathing ending with gasping, snoring, or choking sounds. Often OSA and OSH are grouped together in the diagnosis of obstructive sleep apnea, because they both last ten seconds or longer, causing a decrease in blood oxygen, typically 4%, but in severe cases, 20%-40% or more. They cause frequent but brief arousals from sleep (which the patient does not remember) and sleep deprivation. OSH and OSA induced sleep deprivation usually is associated with the patient obtaining less deep sleep and dream sleep, which seem to be primarily responsible for mental and physical renewal and healing affects of sleep. Not enough deep sleep and dream sleep, as well as interrupted sleep, apparently cause an increase in excessive daytime sleepiness. Both OSA and OSH require treatment as discussed later.

Not all breathing noise during sleep is snoring. A high-pitched sound or even a barking noise may mean that the source of the noise is in the area of the larynx or voice box. If these noises come on suddenly, continue after the person has awakened, or if there is shortness of breath, then this is not simply snoring. Anyone with these symptoms should seek medical attention.

Most Snorers Do Not Have Obstructive Sleep Apnea

Snoring always occurs with obstructive sleep apnea. When diagnosing sleep disorders, OSA is excluded if snoring is not a symptom. All snorers do not necessarily have sleep apnea, but they may have OSH or UARS. However, because they almost certainly have some physical obstruction in their airways, they may develop sleep apnea.

Snoring—Sounding an Alarm

Our bodies were created with a built-in alarm system. Snoring is an alarm that signals something is not functioning quite right within the nasal and/or throat airway of the snorer. Snoring that is loud, erratic, disruptive, and accompanied by EDS should be taken seriously. Such snoring and symptoms may be a signal that the person could have OSA.

Anyone whose snoring is loud and erratic should see their primary care physician or a sleep specialist as soon as possible. Primary care physicians can refer patients to sleep specialists.

Chapter 4

SLEEP APNEA: THE LIFE-THREATENING DISEASE

A well-known sleep apnea "patient" in literature is Charles Dickens' fictional character, Fat Joe, in *The Posthumous Papers of the Pickwick Club.* Fat Joe was the overweight, red-faced boy in a permanent state of sleepiness, snoring and breathing heavily. The term "Pickwickian Syndrome" has been used to describe patients with the most severe form of sleep apnea associated with reduced levels of breathing, even during the day.

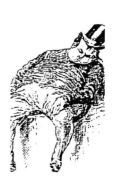

What is Sleep Apnea?

From the Greek word *apnea,* meaning "want of breath," OSA is a serious, potentially life-threatening condition that is far more common than generally understood. First isolated in 1965, OSA is a breathing disorder characterized by brief interruptions of breathing during sleep.

An "apnea" is defined as an absence of air flow for 10 seconds or more. A person with a typical case of sleep apnea will have apneas (breathing pauses) that last 10 to 60 seconds or longer and will experience 20 to 30 apneic events per hour during sleep. During an apnea, the airway becomes blocked and no air flows between the tissues in the throat.

There are three types of sleep apnea: obstructive, central, and mixed. Obstructive sleep apnea, or OSA, is the more common form of the syndrome, which occurs when air cannot flow into or out of the person's nose or mouth. This obstruction of air flow is due to structures in the throat blocking the flow of air in and out of the lungs during sleep although efforts to breathe continue. Central sleep apnea (CSA) occurs when the brain fails to send the appropriate signals to the breathing muscles to initiate respiration, in a sense "forgetting" to breathe during sleep. Mixed sleep apnea (MSA) is a combination of both OSA and CSA.

In any given night the number of involuntary breathing pauses or "apneic events" in a sufferer of OSA may be as low as five per hour to cause daytime sleepiness, but often are as high as 30 or more per hour. Researchers report that among 35 OSA patients studied at Stanford University's Sleep Disorders Clinic, apneic episodes ranged between 68 and an amazing 682 times during seven-hour sleep studies. The length of each apneic episode lasted between 10 and 190 seconds. These breathing pauses are almost always accompanied by snoring between episodes. OSA can also be characterized by choking and suffocation during sleep.

A study of 12 persons suffering from sleep apnea revealed that their sleep was very agitated, and frequently they moved around in an abnormal manner before they resumed breathing at the end of the apneic period. The movements ranged from simple "flapping tremors" of the hands and feet to larger and sometimes quite violent movements of the arms, legs, or even the entire body. Some individuals would suddenly sit up in bed, try to get out of bed and often succeed—try to walk, walk a little, and then fall to the floor where they often would sleep for the rest of the night. All of these people were difficult to awaken during apneic episodes, and if suddenly awakened, they did not know where they were.

What Happens in an OSA Episode

Certain mechanical and structural problems in the airway cause the interruptions in breathing during sleep. In some people, apnea occurs when the throat muscles and tongue relax during sleep and partially block the opening of the airway. When the muscles of the soft palate, the tongue, and the uvula relax and sag, the airway becomes blocked, making breathing labored and noisy, sometimes stopping it altogether. OSA can occur in obese people when an excessive amount of tissue in the airway causes it to be narrowed. The person continues to struggle to breathe, snoring heavily, stopping breathing and experiencing frequent arousals (typically abrupt awakening from light sleep or dream sleep).

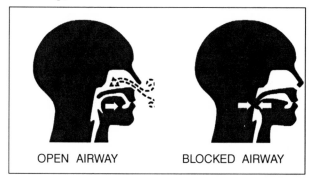

OPEN AIRWAY   BLOCKED AIRWAY

The arousals occur when an imbalance of blood gases, namely a lack of oxygen and an increased level of carbon dioxide (due to its not being exhaled properly) occurs. The brain sends a signal to the upper airway muscles to open the airway, and breathing usually resumes, often with a large snort or gasp. These frequent arousals, although necessary for breathing to restart, prevent the patient from getting enough restorative deep sleep. Ingestion of alcohol and sleeping pills increases the frequency, duration, and intensity of breathing pauses in people with OSA.

Researchers have shown that serious abnormalities of the heart and blood vessels result from continued apneic episodes. The blood pressure rises sharply in both the pulmonary and systemic arteries and the heart slows (bradycardia) and may stop entirely (asystole) for as long as six to eight seconds. These changes are temporarily reversed when breathing is resumed.

The Negative Effects of Sleep Apnea

The consequences of sleep apnea range from simply annoying to life-threatening. Because of the serious disturbances in their normal sleep patterns, people with OSA often feel very sleepy during the day and their concentration and daytime performance suffer. They can also suffer from depression, irritability, sexual dysfunction, learning and memory difficulties, and falling asleep at inappropriate times. There can be a decrease in sexual desire, and bed-wetting occurs frequently in both children and adult sufferers.

Many people with this condition also suffer from high blood pressure. A report by The National Sleep Foundation stated that it has been recently shown that sleep apnea contributes to high blood pressure. Risk for heart attacks and stroke may also increase in those with sleep apnea.

The National Center For Sleep Disorders Research at the National Institute of Health has sponsored a $14 million study that will attempt to define precisely the link between sleep apnea and high blood pressure, heart attack, stroke, and other cardiovascular diseases.

The National Commission on Sleep Disorders Research reports that, in terms of mortality and morbidity, the most serious sleep disorder is OSA. The Commission estimates that *38,000 cardiovascular deaths due to sleep apnea occur annually.* Individuals with untreated OSA are seven times more likely to have automobile accidents than others.

Dangers of Letting OSA Go Untreated

Sleep apnea is a serious disorder that robs its victims of restful sleep and may cause considerable health problems. It can decrease the quality of life for anyone who goes untreated. When left untreated, the disorder can lead to serious consequences such as: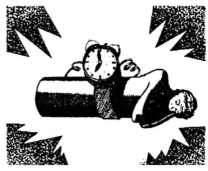

- Increased risk of heart problems
- Increased risk of stroke
- Increased risk of high blood pressure
- Motor vehicle accidents or accidents at work
- Death

When OSA is untreated, it is like a time bomb ticking away, waiting to explode.

Coexisting Diseases

OSA can be life-threatening. People with OSA have a higher risk of serious health problems like diabetes, high blood pressure, heart disease, stroke, and obesity.
Treating OSA can improve these conditions, as well as a person's overall quality of life.

Diabetes

Approximately 60% of Type 2 patients with diabetes have OSA. Studies have shown that sleep apnea contributes to insulin resistance, which can lead to Type 2 diabetes. Patients with diabetes who receive treatment for OSA have been shown to experience an immediate improvement in their diabetic condition. Treating OSA can help patients with diabetes control their blood sugar levels and may lower their risk of complications such as heart disease.

High Blood Pressure

The National Institutes of Health (NIH) lists sleep apnea as a cause of high blood pressure. Approximately 35% of all people with high blood pressure have OSA. That number increases to 80% for people taking three or more medications for their uncontrolled blood pressure. OSA patients with high blood pressure can reduce their levels significantly by receiving OSA treatment. OSA treatment has been shown to reduce blood pressure and improve heart function.

Heart Disease

Untreated OSA puts prolonged stress on the heart and has a negative impact on heart function in general. It can lead to high blood pressure, irregular heartbeat, and stroke. Left untreated, OSA contributes to heart disease and heart failure. These risk factors may be improved with treatment. People who receive treatment for OSA are able to control their blood pressure and improve the overall function of their heart and vascular system.

Stroke

OSA can increase a person's risk of stroke. In fact, more than 60% of patients who have had a stroke also have OSA. Stroke patients with OSA are at a major disadvantage during recovery from stroke. Recovering from a stroke takes sustained energy and motivation, but the sleepiness and fatigue caused by OSA can make it difficult for a person to follow rehabilitation programs, resulting in poor recovery. Stroke patients with untreated OSA have higher mortality rates post-stroke than others do.

Obesity

OSA affects up to 40% of obese people. Overweight people with OSA should be particularly concerned because OSA makes weight loss more difficult. The sleepiness caused by OSA may cause people to overeat, sleep more, and exercise less. Some people, as a matter of habit, will eat to "wake up" when they feel drowsy during the day. That in turn causes them to gain more weight, which makes OSA even worse. Being treated for OSA can help obese people gain the energy to exercise more and lose weight. Additionally, weight loss has been shown to improve OSA for some obese patients.

OSA and Sudden Infant Death Syndrome

Sleep apnea is sometimes implicated in sudden infant death syndrome (SIDS), also called crib death. About 10,000 infants die every year in this country from SIDS. Scientists have not yet reached a conclusion for the reason for these deaths, but sleep apnea may play a role, because the babies die when they are asleep and show no evidence of trauma. On autopsy, pinpoint hemorrhages are sometimes noted in the thoracic cavity, which may be caused by lack of oxygen prior to cardiac arrest and vigorous respiratory movements. "Wake Up, America: A National Sleep Alert" reveals the following information concerning sleep in infants:

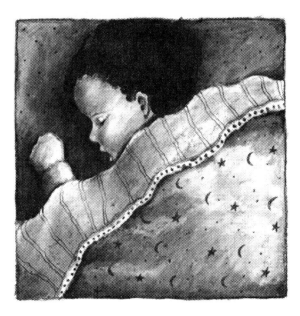

In the United States, two of every 1,000 babies born will die from sudden infant death syndrome (SIDS). SIDS claims more lives between the ages of one month and one year than all other causes of death combined. SIDS is linked inextricably to sleep; more than 70% of its victims are found in the early morning hours after the nighttime sleep. While a number of theories have been proposed to explain the mechanisms of SIDS, none has received unequivocal substantiation.

SIDS: "Back to Sleep" Campaign

The National Institute of Child Health & Human Development (NICHD) states that the "Back to Sleep" campaign is suitably named for its recommendation to place healthy babies on their backs to sleep. Placing babies on their backs to sleep reduces the risk of SIDS. This campaign has been successful in promoting infant back sleeping to parents, family members, child care providers, health professionals, and all other care givers of infants.

This campaign is sponsored by the NICHD, the Maternal and Child Health Bureau, the American Academy of Pediatrics, the SIDS Alliance, and the Association of SIDS and Infant Mortality Program.

OSA in Children

OSA can also occur in children who snore. If your child snores, you should discuss it with your child's doctor or healthcare provider.

In preschool-age children, the most obvious symptom of sleep apnea is typically failure to thrive (shorter and/or underweight). Older children may seem sluggish and often perform poorly in school. Sometimes they are labeled "slow" or "lazy."

More boys than girls develop sleep apnea. It is also more common in those who are overweight. Children with sleep apnea may snore, squeak, appear to have difficulty breathing, or sleep fitfully. It is not normal for children to snore. Parents should bring a child's nighttime noise to a doctor's attention and a board-certified sleep specialist.

In children, OSA is thought to impair learning ability and increase behavioral problems due to increased daytime sleepiness, masquerading as hyperactivity, since sleepy children tend to counter sleepiness by moving around.

OSA in Adolescents

According to researchers, this age group is when snoring/OSA is mostly likely to start. It's a time when young people are much more active in school, sports, and part-time jobs. This is also a time when many teenagers start driving automobiles. Sleepiness due to OSA can affect a youngster's development and school performance. In addition to placing young people at high risk for automobile crashes, problem sleepiness can impair learning, perceptual skills, and memory, which may lead to poor school performance and grades.

In adolescents and young adults, mood, attention, and behavior deteriorate when they obtain inadequate sleep. These changes may interfere with a teenager's ability to cope with daily stressors.

Parents and guardians should be on the look out for behavioral changes in young people. If the youngster snores, this red flag signals some airway obstructions may be causing the snoring. Adults should take adolescents to a doctor as soon as possible.

Combating Sleep Attacks on the Job Due to OSA

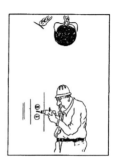

I suffered the most with excessive daytime sleepiness (EDS). Sleep attacks would hit me mainly during the afternoons, especially after lunch. It would strike when I sat down or drove, but as long as I stood and moved about, I was all right. It was a struggle for me to keep awake and alert at work.

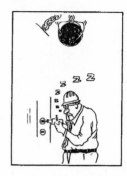

I recall many times I would be working at my desk at the office and feel myself get drowsy and begin to nod. Routinely I would get up and wash my face in the men's room to get rid of the sleepiness. Other times, if I felt really sleepy, I would go outside for a short walk and some fresh air.

I always wanted to present my best image at work, especially at company meetings. But because I suffered with EDS, company meetings presented a challenge for me.

Resisting Sleep Attacks While Driving Due to OSA

In addition to fighting EDS at the office, I faced the same challenge while driving home from work. It was an enormous struggle to stay alert while driving home on the busy freeways. It was frightening to hear another driver's horn and realize I had drifted too close to another car. It was scary to be stopped at a traffic light and feel myself starting to dose off, or become startled awake by the horns of the irate drivers behind me. These experiences were a source of embarrassment and fear. However, the main problem for a person hit with a sleep attack while driving, of course, is the extreme danger of causing a crash.

People tend to fall asleep on high-speed, long, or rural highways. (For example, New York Police estimate that 30% of all fatal crashes along the New York Thruway occurred because the driver fell asleep at the wheel.)

I am relieved to report that, in spite of my EDS and some near car accidents, I was able to maintain an accident-free driving record and my job performance remained high.

Danger Signs of a Fatigued and Drowsy Driver

Before treatment for OSA, I generally could tell when I was about to fall asleep; however, sometimes you may not be aware of being fatigued or drowsy. If you experience any of the following danger signs while driving, take them as a warning that you could fall asleep without meaning to.

1. Your eyelids begin to feel heavy and tired.
2. Your eyes close or go out of focus by themselves.
3. Your head bobs by itself.
4. You can't stop yawning.
5. You can't focus on a complete thought.
6. You doze off while stopped at a traffic light.
7. You don't remember driving the last few miles.
8. You drift too close to another vehicle, tail gate, miss a traffic sign, or run a red light.
9. You find it difficult to keep in your traffic lane.

If you have any one of these danger signs, you may fall asleep and cause a crash. Find a safe place to stop, preferably a well-lit rest stop or truck stop. The busier the place you stop to rest, the less opportunity for crime. Always lock all the doors and roll up the windows, turn the engine off, and take a brief nap.

Sound Advice

My ultimate advice to those suffering from EDS is to seek medical attention without delay. When I was tested for loud snoring and EDS, the treatment prescribed for me was the Continuous Positive Airway Pressure (CPAP). Faithful use has stopped my snoring, OSA, and EDS.

Other sleep disorders, such as insomnia and narcolepsy, are known to cause fragmented sleep, which results in EDS. If you suspect you have a sleep problem, consult your primary care physician or arrange a consultation with a sleep disorders specialist, certified by the American Board of Sleep Medicine (ABSM). Visit www.sleepcenters.org for a listing of certified sleep centers in your area. These sleep centers have sleep specialists on their staff available for consultation.

Did Snoring Cause NFL Hall of Famer, Reggie White's Death?

Football is my favorite sport and I was a huge fan of Reggie White's superstar performance on the football field; but I also greatly admired Reggie White's ministry off the field. So I'm pleased to offer my sincere congratulations to Mr. White's wife, Sara, on his induction into the Pro. Football Hall of Fame.

Autopsy Report

Reggie White died at the age of 43 on the morning of December 26, 2004. His autopsy report revealed that he was found unresponsive while sleeping in his bed. Prior to his unresponsiveness, there was reportedly 'snoring' followed by respiratory distress. The autopsy further revealed that Mr. White had a history of sleep apnea and other complications including sarcoidosis.

A U.S. newswire article released on December 29, 2004, titled *"Famous Athlete, Reggie White, Dies from Complications of Untreated Sleep Apnea,"* stated: "The untimely and tragic death last weekend of National Football League legend, Reggie White serves as a warning of the grave consequences of untreated sleep apnea, which is reported to have contributed in part to White's death."

Obstructive sleep apnea is a very common sleep disorder which not only has a debilitating effect on sleep, but it is also detrimental to one's overall health and quality of life."

"Mr. White's premature and sad death is a mournful reminder of the toll that is taken by this prevalent condition," said Michael J. Sateia, M.D., president of the American Academy of Sleep Medicine (AASM) and medical director of The Sleep Center at Darmouth-Hitchcock Medical Center. He further stated, "This disorder is readily treatable."

Chapter 5

ASSESSING POTENTIAL SLEEP DISORDERS AND SELF-HELP TREATMENTS

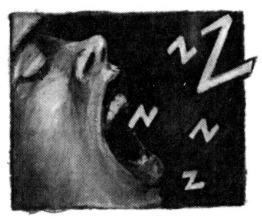

Snorer's First Line Responders

I believe spouses, family members, friends, roommates, and coworkers are in a unique position to help identify a loved one or friend who shows symptoms of OSA. Therefore I have designated the mates, family members, friends, roommates, and coworkers of a person who snores loudly as the Snorer's First Line Responders (SFLR).

The SFLR may share the same bed, household, or bunk in the same firehouse with the person who snores, and their actions could actually help their love one or friend live longer and healthier. Sleep apnea is a life-threatening disease when left untreated, therefore the SFLR can in fact save a life.

Most often, people who snore and have OSA do not know

the extent of their snoring and they do not know that they have OSA. They are not aware that their breathing stops and starts many times while they sleep.

I admit that, although I had been told countless times (over the years) of my loud, erratic snoring, it did not hit home until I heard a recording of my snoring. Then I understood why everyone else was making so much fuss about my snoring.

What Can Family Members and Friends Do To Help

Since family members, roommates, and bed partners are usually the first ones to notice that the person snores and stops breathing while sleeping, the author has added a SFLR Quiz to this fourth edition.

Snorer's First Line Responder's Quiz

The questions below are to be completed by a SFLR. Does your mate, family member, friend, roommate, or co-worker show any of the following markers and/or symptoms?

1. Yes____No____ Snore loudly?
2. Yes____No____ Stop breathing during sleep?
3. Yes____No____ Awaken gasping or short of breath?
4. Yes____No____ Have high blood pressure?
5. Yes____No____ Experience excessive daytime sleepiness?
6. Yes____No____ Have congestive heart failure?
7. Yes____No____ Lack concentration or have memory lapses?
8. Yes____No____ Overweight?
9. Yes____No____ Decreased interest in sex?
10. Yes____No____ Man's neck size 17 or larger, woman's neck size 16 or larger?
11. Yes____No____ Have little or no dreams?
12. Yes____No____ Fall asleep in less than five minutes?

If you marked yes to question #1, and yes to at least another question, then it is your duty as the SFLR to select an appropriate time to sit down for a sincere talk with your loved one or friend. This discussion should be conducted in an atmosphere of concern and caring and not in a critical way. When sharing the results of the quiz, the SFLR should encourage in a kind way the loved one or friend to make an appointment and see their primary care physician or a board certified sleep specialist as soon as possible. Don't be afraid to offer to make the appointment for the person who snores.

Should the person who snores not follow through and see a doctor, then the SFLR should move to Plan B which is the SFLR Snoring Assessment Study.

SFLR Snoring Assessment Study

This simple and easy Snoring Assessment Study is primarily for use by the SFLR. However the person who snores can conduct this study, especially those individuals who live alone. It is designed to reveal how loud, how erratic, how obnoxious, and how long an individual snores during the night. And the purpose of this study is to help convince the snorer of the severity of her/his sleep problem.

(This study is not to be substituted for a certified sleep center's sleep evaluation.)

As has already been stated, snoring can be extremely hazardous to your health. Because of this, the SFLR should be well informed of the snorer's sleep activities, including the person's sleep position, whether the snoring is only when the person is lying on his back. Or does the person snore when sleeping on her side? If the person sleeps on her stomach, does the snoring stop? When a person snores on his back and on his side, he generally is dubbed an obnoxious snorer.

Here is how you begin this test:

Step 1: For three nights use a voice-activated tape recorder to tape yourself as you sleep. Use three 100- or 90-minute audio or micro cassette tapes, one for each night. These tapes provide longer monitoring time. Place the recorder on your bedside table and set it to the record mode. Speak the date and time into the recorder.

Step 2: Set up three columns on a sheet of paper, (your Snoring Assessment Sheet), labeling the columns *Night One, Night Two,* and *Night Three.* Log your bedtime in the appropriate column each night.

Step 3: If you awaken during the night, check the recorder to see if more than 1/2 hour of the tape has been used. If so, make a notation on the tape of the time, then fast-forward the tape to the end, flip it over to the other side and reset. Note the time in the appropriate column on the Snoring Assessment Sheet, plus speak the time into the recorder, then resume sleep.

Step 4: When you awaken each morning, record the time on your Snore Assessment Sheet. Be sure to listen carefully to the complete tape each morning and keep track of the amount of time used up on the tape.

Step 5: After the third night of taping, add the total number of hours you slept, then add the total time that was recorded on the three cassettes.

Step 6: If you record more than 30 minutes of snoring each night and/or detect loud, erratic snoring, snorting, or quiet pauses ending with a gasp or uneven snoring or breathing, then I recommend that you contact your physician or an accredited sleep disorders center to arrange for consultation with a sleep specialist. Be sure to take your Snoring Assessment Sheet, the tapes, and your SFLR quiz with you so your physician or sleep specialist can evaluate the information.

This SFLR Snoring Assessment Study is designed to highlight symptoms associated with OSA. *It is intended as a general source of educational information only and does not contain medical advice. It should not be used for self-diagnosis or treatment.* Only a sleep evaluation made at a sleep center under the direction of an experienced staff with expertise in sleep medicine can determine if you have a specific sleep disorder.

The Sleep Questionnaire
Do you, or does a family member, have a sleep problem? These questions are designed primarily for the snorer. All answers will come in a "yes" or "no" form.

1. Yes____ No____ Does anyone complain about your snoring?
2. Yes____ No____ Do you awaken with a sore throat or dry mouth and throat?
3. Yes____ No____ Do you experience excessive daytime sleepiness?
4. Yes____ No____ Do you awaken with morning head aches, fatigue, or grogginess?
5. Yes____ No____ Does anyone report to you that you stop breathing, gasp for air, or make choking sounds while sleeping?
6. Yes____ No____ Do you awaken with lightheadedness?
7. Yes____ No____ Have you been diagnosed with high blood pressure?
8. Yes____ No____ Do you need multiple naps?
9. Yes____ No____ Is your blood pressure only elevated in the morning?
10. Yes____ No____ Does anyone complain of your excessive movement while sleeping?
11. Yes____ No____ Do you drowse while driving?
12. Yes____ No____ Is your collar size 17 or larger? (Woman's neck size 16 or larger?)

13. Yes____ No____ Has anyone mentioned to you that you snore when you sleep on your back and on your side?
14. Yes____ No____ Are you forgetful?
15. Yes____ No____ Do you drowse at inappropriate times (at work, public places or events)?
16. Yes____ No____ Have you had episodes of hallucination?
17. Yes____ No____ Are you fatigued regardless of how many hours you have slept?
18. Yes____ No____ Have you experienced episodes of bed-wetting?
19. Yes____ No____ Are you overweight?
20. Yes____ No____ Have you noticed a diminished sex drive?

If you answered Yes to question #1 and three other questions, then you show markers and/or symptoms of OSA, and you should urgently discuss your symptoms with your physician or arrange a consultation with a sleep specialist, board-certified by the American Board of Sleep Medicine, which may involve an overnight sleep study. If you are excessively sleepy, a daytime nap test called the Multiple Sleep Latency Test should be considered. Test results should be interpreted by a qualified sleep specialist. Be sure to take this questionnaire with you so the physician or specialist can evaluate the information.

This questionnaire is designed to inform you of symptoms that may indicate a problem with OSA. It is intended as a general source of educational information and does not contain medical advice, and should not be used for the purpose of self-diagnosis or unassisted treatment. Only a sleep evaluation at a sleep center with an experienced staff having expertise in sleep medicine can determine whether or not you have a specific sleep disorder.

The good news is that when people hear how loud and erratic their snoring is they are more likely to do something about getting help.

That's what happened with me—the first time I heard myself on audiotape, I was fully persuaded that I had a major problem. I didn't like what I heard. For over four decades, I had been unaware of how I sounded when I slept. Although many individuals in my family (including some youngsters) have mimicked my snoring accurately, I didn't realize until I heard the tape that my snoring pattern was very abnormal. I immediately made an appointment to see my doctor and employed some self-help remedies such as daily exercise and sleeping on my side. My doctor scheduled me for a sleep study.

My desire for you is that after this Sleep Questionnaire is conducted, it will prompt the person who snores to make an appointment with his primary care physician or a board certified sleep specialist for consultation and possible sleep study. On your appointment to the doctor, be sure to take along the answers to the SFLR Quiz, the Sleep Questionnaire, and your Snoring Assessment Study tapes.

Chapter 6

SELF-HELP METHODS TO STOP SNORING AND OSA

Doctors, like all of us, have certain preferences about one thing or another. Most doctors are highly trained and skillful in their profession and dedicated to quality patient care.

However, I have found that depending upon which specialist (pulmonary, otolaryngologist, or dentist) you talk with about treatment for snoring and OSA, you will probably get a response that leans favorably toward the treatment which that doctor provides (CPAP, surgery, or oral appliances).

When patients are unaware of other treatment options or do not know what specific questions to ask the doctor concerning treatment options, they are sometimes readily influenced by the first doctor they see and agree to the treatment which that doctor provides.

I believe everyone benefits when the patient is fully aware of all the treatment options available for snoring/OSA.

Therefore, I strongly recommend that individuals who are concerned about their sleep problem should contact their primary care physician and request a consultation with a board-certified sleep specialist. The patient should ask the sleep specialist questions about treatment options for snoring/OSA, including questions about the treatment's risk, benefits, compliance record, success rate, complications/side effects, cost, and long-term record in prevention of death and disability.

Also, for a good source of patient-awareness information, I recommend that individuals who are concerned about a sleep problem should contact a local sleep center to find out if there is a patient advocacy group in their area. You may also contact the national office of A.W.A.K.E. (Alert, Well, and Keeping Energetic). It is a network of hundreds of mutual-help support groups throughout the United States for persons effected by sleep apnea. Call the network support group at (202) 293-3650 to find the location of an A.W.A.K.E. group in your area.

Be sure to find out as much as possible about the different treatment options for snoring/OSA. Patients attending the A.W.A.K.E. meeting can speak of their personal experiences with sleep disorders, diagnosis process, treatment, and learn valuable information from other patients.

Position Therapy: Stay Off Your Back

For ages, snorers have received a jab in the ribs as a reminder to roll over and stop snoring. It's true, snoring is worsened with back sleeping. That's because gravity is at work to open the mouth, allowing the tongue to move backwards into the throat, blocking airflow. It's easier to keep the mouth closed when sleeping on one's side.

Basic snoring (at best) can be disruptive to a peaceful family life. Therefore, for everyone involved, it's advisable to use any working method to combat this robber of a full night's sleep. For some individuals who snore and in mild cases of sleep apnea, breathing pauses occur only when the individual sleeps on his back. Thus, using position therapy methods that will ensure patients sleep on their side is often helpful. In such cases, using a tennis ball sewn into the pajama back, or the "Backstopper," a specially designed four-inch lightweight ball, should help keep the snorer off his back. When the ball is placed in the right position, the snorer becomes uncomfortable when he rolls over on his back. This encourages the snorer to sleep on his stomach or side. I place the

Backstopper in an athletic sock and attach it to the back of my pajama top. The sock should be positioned in the middle of the back. More severe snorers will make gasping sounds in all positions, prone, right, left, and back. Patients with these symptoms should seek an evaluation with a board-certified sleep disorder specialist as soon as possible.

Proper Humidification Aids

Using vaporizers and humidifiers will help put moisture into the air, keeping the nasal tract free from drying out and becoming congested. This not only makes breathing easier, it helps to prevent nasal obstructions due to dryness, thereby alleviating dryness-caused snoring. It can also combat susceptibility to respiratory disease. In addition the whole family benefits when the air is properly humidified. Do not let water sit in the humidifier during the day, since bacteria will grow and could promote infections.

Behavioral Changes Are Essential: Weight Loss, Avoid Alcohol and Tobacco, Certain Medications

Behavioral changes are an important part of the treatment program, and in mild cases, behavioral therapy may be all that is needed. The individual should avoid the use of alcohol, tobacco, sleeping pills, and other medications that cause drowsiness. These make the airway susceptible to collapse during sleep, prolonging the apneic periods. In addition, regular exercise and proper diet with reduction of fat intake are great steps toward improving one's health. Overweight people can benefit from losing weight. Even a 10% weight loss can help reduce snoring and the number of apneic events for most OSA patients. However, weight loss tends to be very difficult when you are excessively sleepy. Successful treatment of OSA and hypopnea, which cause excessive sleepiness, will allow you to lose weight more easily.

My snoring problem was exacerbated because I was overweight. I encourage anyone who is more than 20% over the average weight for his/her age, sex, and height, to discuss weight loss through dieting and an exercise plan with a physician.

Substance Involvement and Its Link with Snoring

Research reveals that drinking alcohol in the evening increases the frequency and severity of obstructive sleep apnea/hypopnea and snoring during sleep.

Alcohol usage reduces muscle tone in the throat tissues when a person is asleep. The tissue becomes relaxed and more flabby, and the swift movement of air in the throat causes the snoring.

Sleeping pills depress breathing and promote erratic breathing and snoring. Coffee and other stimulants, such as certain decongestant medicines, can negatively affect people who have various degrees of sensitivity to such substances. Some find they can't drink coffee after noon without having their sleep disrupted many hours later. It's advisable to check cold and allergy medications for ingredients that may cause wakefulness.

A number of studies have concluded that smoking increases the risk of snoring, possibly because smoking causes inflammation in the throat. One study suggests that a smoking history may be a risk factor proportionate to the amount of tobacco used.

Avoiding heavy meals after 6 p.m. may lessen snoring attacks. The extra load on your stomach and upper respiratory system aggravates breathing and promotes snoring. It is much better to eat your largest meal around noon.

Developing a Healthier Positive Attitude

The hallmark of most notable people has been to set goals in every aspect of their lives, then go about working to achieve their goals. Setting goals aimed at improving health should be a top priority.

The desire to learn more about snoring and my positive outlook toward finding a cure resulted in my accomplishing both goals. I completed a job-related motivational course in 1982. This training helped me to see myself and others in a better perspective. I found out it requires the same amount of energy and effort to form bad attitudes as it does to form good attitudes.

I wrote some positive statements about every aspect of my life and repeated those statements aloud numerous times each day. Four of my daily affirmations were, "I believe I now get a good night's sleep. I do not snore. I sleep well. I feel good the next day." I can now say that these affirmations and others have been fulfilled. I firmly believe that "You are what you say all day long."

Chapter 7

PHYSICIAN-PRESCRIBED TREATMENTS TO STOP SNORING AND OSA

The Oximeter: A Useful Device Used to Screen for OSA

Dr. Lawrence E. Kline has been my sleep specialist since 1998, and he has prescribed the oximetery study for me many times. The purpose of this study is to give your doctor a report of how well you breathe during sleep. The study measures oxygen levels in the body during sleep.

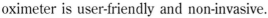

For this study an oximeter, a device about the size of an I-pod with a thin cable, is attached to a finger probe. The oximeter is user-friendly and non-invasive.

When Dr. Kline prescribes this study for me, he will issue me an oximeter and provide the simple instructions to follow, which includes a brief bedtime questionnaire and a morning questionnaire.

When I'm ready for bed, I complete the bedtime questionnaire, then attach the finger probe by inserting my index or middle finger into the sensor until the end of my finger reaches the stop. Then I turn the oximeter on and place it on the nightstand. Next I put my APAP mask on which automatically turns the APAP machine on, and I'm now ready for sleep.

During the night if I need to make a restroom visit, I simply remove my APAP mask and take the oximeter with me.

When I awaken in the morning, I remove my APAP mask, turn the oximeter off, disconnect the probe, and complete the morning questionnaire. I'm required to return the oximeter to my doctor's pulmonary lab before noon the same day.

At the lab, my sleep data on the oximeter is downloaded and a printout is given to Dr. Kline who analyzes the data and writes his report. He discusses the results with me, and I always request a copy of the study data and his report for my home files.

The doctor decides whether additional tests are needed and if the PAP system air pressure is adequate.

The oximetery study is also valuable in screening the new patients for OSA.

The Doctor's Comments

Dr. Kline said the following about the oximetery test:

Oxygen in the blood can be measured now with a simple device that measures adsorption of light. The hemoglobin in blood binds to oxygen causing the color of blood to change to a brighter red. The oximetry test needs at least two different light wavelengths to derive the oxygen saturation. Technology has allowed the development of a probe, usually placed on the finger, that can be applied on the skin and deliver the light beam while recording which wavelengths are adsorbed. These probes are as small as Band-Aids or clothespins and require no needles. This gives us a reasonably accurate measurement of the level of oxygen in the blood which can vary in a wide range of conditions including sleep apnea.

The saturation of oxygen in hemoglobin refers to the percent of hemoglobin bound to oxygen compared to the total amount of hemoglobin available for binding. The saturation of blood as it enters the lungs is 75% since it comes from the body after the oxygen has been extracted or used. A normal saturation in a healthy person in the arterial system where blood is pumped after it comes out of the lungs should be approximately 95%. This measurement may vary as much as 4% up or down under normal conditions.

If we can take moments in time and record the oxygen level or saturation in the arterial circulation we can see a useful pattern. The frequency the microprocessor of the oximeter detects and records saturation can greatly influence the result. If the detection frequency is once a minute, even fluctuations that happen in 10 to 15 seconds can be missed. Most good devices have sampling intervals at least every 3 to 5 seconds. This allows us to see a drop in oxygen that might occur if an apnea or under breathing period causes it and results in this change.

The use of oxygen saturation recordings are common in doctors' offices and hospitals. These measurements reveal a numerical saturation and may vary over time. Many of these devices do not record saturations with the sampling interval of 3 to 5 seconds and later print a tracing. The printing of the saturation recording over time allows an analysis of the pattern of saturation. This can be a useful tool to screen for sleep apnea.

A normal saturation recording does not exclude the diagnosis of sleep apnea because some apneas interrupt sleep without causing a drop in saturation. If however there are fluctuations in the saturation of more than 4% in a cohesive pattern, the oximetry can be helpful in suggesting sleep apnea. Therefore an abnormal test helps, but a normal test does not exclude the diagnosis.

Physician-Prescribed Treatment: CPAP Devices that Stop Snoring, OSH, and OSA

The device known as Continuous Positive Airway Pressure (CPAP) is the most effective non-invasive therapy for OSA. CPAP is the best, safest, and quickest treatment for snoring, OSH, and OSA. Researchers indicate that the physiological results of CPAP treatment are 95% successful in the laboratory, and 50-85% successful in long-term adherence to CPAP therapy. CPAP therapy has a proven track record in the treatment of OSA and is well documented in hundreds of medical publications.

The CPAP system is a mechanical device which can be placed on a bedside table. A flexible tube runs from the device to a mask which is placed on the patient's nose during the time of normal sleep.

The CPAP system has a fan that moves air through the tube to the mask. The air pressure is set inside the device to fit the patient's own breathing pattern.

The patient wears a sealed mask over the nose or, in some cases, over the nose and mouth during sleep. The mask is connected to a blower which forces air through the nasal passages. The CPAP acts like a cushion of air by increasing the pressure in the upper airway, thereby maintaining an open airway throughout the ventilatory cycle. The cushion of air supports the soft tissues in the upper airway of the mouth and throat and prevents the tissues from being drawn closer together (causing snoring) or collapsing together (causing OSA).

The CPAP system works to prevent tissues in the throat from blocking air movement in and out of the lungs. This is accomplished with small amounts of air pressure applied through the nose. The pressure works to keep the airway open, which allows air to move from the nose to the top of the patient's windpipe (trachea).

When air is able to move freely in and out of the throat airway and into the lungs, the patient will have enough oxygen and the patient's sleep will no longer be disturbed by receiving too little oxygen.

The treatment is prescribed after a polysomnogram (overnight sleep study) has first determined the therapeutic level of CPAP pressure required to reduce or eliminate OSA.

The CPAP system is safe; it cannot be accidentally adjusted to levels other than what the doctor ordered. In case of an electrical power failure or should the patient displace the mask during sleep, the patient will continue to breathe through the mouth as he usually does. According to sleep specialists, a trial of CPAP should be considered as the first step in the treatment of OSA.

CPAP is effective in reversing EDS. When properly used, it produces normal breathing, resulting in the patient's feeling dramatically better and able to function more efficiently. It is used as a technique for patients whose breathing is impaired to the point that their carbon dioxide levels are elevated, as happens in obesity-hypoventilation syndrome and certain neuromuscular diseases. Compared with non-treatment or other treatments, patients using CPAP have been shown to have a lower mortality rate.

CPAP usually causes immediate cessation of snoring, gasping and choking sounds, when it is adjusted to the appropriate pressure level. The appropriate pressure level is best obtained by spending a second night in the sleep laboratory which allows enough time to test several pressure settings so that at each pressure some REM sleep occurs. The most severe OSH and OSA usually occur during REM sleep. Excessive daytime sleepiness is also improved quickly by CPAP, usually within several days or a few weeks. If excessive sleepiness persists despite using CPAP, then the CPAP pressure setting may not be optimal or there may be other medical problems such as periodic limb movements causing sleep disturbances, or even the use of some medications will cause sleepiness to persist. The board-certified sleep specialist works with your family physician to assess all these possibilities and make appropriate treatment recommendations.

On recommendation from my sleep center study, I was referred to an ENT (ear, nose and throat) specialist, who closely examined my nasal passage, tonsils, soft palate, uvula, tongue, and throat airways for signs of enlargement and blockage. These tissues are the key cause of snoring. The ENT then explained that I had enlarged soft palate and uvula tissue, which were the major causes of my snoring. The ENT said he could trim these tissues surgically, but he could not guarantee the degree of success in reducing the snoring and OSA symptoms. It might have taken a month to fully recover from soreness, and I could have experienced some speech changes after the surgery.

It didn't take me long to make my decision. My next question was whether there were alternatives to surgery. He referred me to a doctor who, upon further evaluation, prescribed a CPAP unit.

How It Feels to Sleep with the CPAP

I have been using a PAP unit successfully for almost two decades. My first experience of sleeping with the CPAP system took place at the Veteran's Administration (VA) Hospital's sleep laboratory. The sleep technician prepared me for a sleep evaluation study, which involved attaching some leads to different parts of my upper body. As I relaxed in bed, he explained that the wires were connected to a polysomnography machine which would monitor, record, and produce a printout of my sleep patterns. He then listed the value of CPAP use, mainly that it is safe to use, should help me sleep more efficiently, and, most importantly, should eliminate my snoring and OSA.

The unit had a headgear and a mask that the technician adjusted to fit my face. I had to adjust my own breathing pattern with the air that was being forced into my nose from the CPAP. In a short time I got the hang of it. Since I was able to move my head freely, the mask and flexible hose didn't bother me much.

When the technician awakened me about four hours later, he informed me that I had fallen asleep in a short time and had slept very well with the CPAP. This encouraged me. The doctor's evaluation confirmed that I showed normal sleep patterns (no OSA) and had not snored during the study. Although this was a good report, I still was not convinced thoroughly that this was all due to the CPAP use.

With the doctor's reassurance, I was issued a CPAP unit for a trial home-use that would last a couple of weeks. She gave me an explanation of the operation and maintenance of the unit, recommending that I initially use the CPAP for two to four hours each night, gradually increasing the time until I was comfortable having the unit operating all night.

The first night at home on the CPAP went well. I set the alarm to awaken me in four hours, turned on my voice-activated cassette recorder, donned the mask, and turned on the CPAP unit. Then I rolled over to my normal right side sleeping position. (I later asked my wife if the sound from the unit had bothered her. She assured me that it was not so loud as to disturb her sleep.)

I awoke to my alarm at 2 a.m. I reached down, eager to rewind the tape to see if I had snored. I had an earlier recording of my snoring without the CPAP, so I was aware of how loud and erratic my nocturnal noises could be. The time for the big test had come, and I was amazed to see that there was very little tape to be rewound. When I played it back, I heard the conversation I had had with my wife prior to our falling asleep. The only other sound on the tape was the alarm that had just awakened me.

Fully persuaded now that the CPAP had stopped my snoring, I was exuberant! This test also proved that the sound of the CPAP was not loud enough to trigger my recorder. Within two weeks I was sleeping all night with my unit, with no side effects.

I have been using a CPAP unit successfully for more than nineteen years. I adapted easily to the system, and rarely sleep without it. I feel great during the day and don't get as sleepy as I did before. My overall outlook on life has become much brighter.

Heading into 2006: Experiences to Date—We've Come a Long Way, Baby!

There has been a gradual improvement over the years in the CPAP therapy devices.

I got my first CPAP system almost two decades ago, and it was rather large, bulky, and noisy. In spite of these factors, this CPAP technology was very effective in preventing snoring and sleep apnea. Then my next CPAP was somewhat smaller, less noisy, and it had a new feature called ramp start. This was a great comfort enhancement, as this feature allowed the CPAP to start out at a very low pressure and gradually increase pressure over a 5, 10, 15, or 30 minute period before reaching the doctor's prescribed pressure setting.

Five years ago, I changed to a new CPAP system, and this unit was smaller than my previous CPAP and it was "library quiet." It was so quiet that often times I would have to rise up and look to see if the light was on, or put my hand in front of my mask to see if air was coming out. It too had the ramp start feature. I got a humidifier with this CPAP, and I was also fitted with a mask that had nasal pillows, both of which provided a lot more comfort.

2006/2007

In the second edition of this book back in 1997, I wrote about a new generation of self-adjusting CPAP systems that would be available in the future. Well, that future is now, and I have what is sometimes referred to as a "smart CPAP." Now, I am using an Auto Positive Airway Pressure (APAP). User-friendly, APAP has a number of excellent features that will be explained later in this chapter. This self-adjusting sleep apnea system has two treatment modes—fixed-pressure CPAP and AutoSet mode. The AutoSet adjusts the air pressure treatment to what you need and when you need it. Therefore the air pressure is not at a continuous setting, but will vary depending on the opening or closing in the throat's airway. Lightweight, it is about half the size of a shoe box. In fact the APAP and its humidifier will fit in a Naturalizer shoe box.

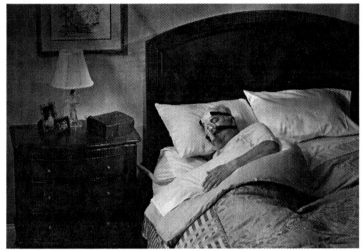

Patient using an M Series REMstar® Pro and a ComfortGel ™ patient mask.

I have found that the APAP provides me with additional convenience and comfort. It is a state-of-the-art system that's a step ahead in the treatment of snoring and sleep apnea. Because it is a self-adjusting system, it may be useful for new patients to help overcome compliance issues, for those who can't tolerate CPAP, or for those who simply want convenience and comfort.

As part of managing your health care, it is wise to ascertain from your insurance carrier what devices or treatments are covered in what percentages.

Drawbacks to CPAP and Solutions

Although very effective, CPAP may be difficult for some

patients to use. Adherence to CPAP treatment varies greatly, but tends to be higher in patients with severe symptoms. The most common reasons for discontinuing CPAP are intolerance of the mask, nasal-related discomfort, and the inconvenience of being connected to a machine. Some people find they cannot tolerate the slightest machine noise. Common side effects include nasal stuffiness, inflamed nasal tissues, facial skin problems, and discomfort with the pressure. These symptoms, however, can often be alleviated with a change of mask type, humidifier attachments, or room humidifiers.

Some doctors also recommend use of nasal steroids or decongestants, intranasal anticholinergics. Switching to a different mask and changing the pressure application have helped patients in improving comfort. It's necessary to obtain help from a professional in determining proper adjustments to increase comfort and adherence to CPAP treatment. The ramp system, a modification of CPAP, is designed to make the treatment more comfortable and allows the pressure to be applied only when the patient achieves sleep, increasing pressure slowly over a 30-minute period.

Some people cannot tolerate CPAP, because of claustrophobic feelings, vanity, and more rarely because of the bed partner's vanity. For married couples, most spouses of the snorer welcome CPAP, which almost cannot be heard when functioning. Tolerance of CPAP has been reported to be as low as 50% and as high as 85% in different reports.

Follow-up Necessary with CPAP

Follow-up after the first month of CPAP treatment should include checking the status of equipment, assessing patient symptoms, and adherence and assessing the status of coexisting conditions such as hypertension. In patients who have achieved significant weight loss, or if the patient continues snoring, the CPAP pressure may need to be adjusted.

For CPAP to work effectively, it must be used nightly. Sometimes when patients have an upper respiratory infection (a cold), they cannot use CPAP, because the nasal passage is blocked. Nasal decongestants can often overcome this temporary problem. After 6 to 12 months' use of CPAP, the patient should be retested to see if they still need CPAP or need it at a different pressure setting. Often patients will lose weight and/or their swollen soft tissue will shrink back—no longer being irritated by the drying and vibrating effects that snoring, OSH, and OSA cause. Usually the CPAP pressure needs to be decreased. In some cases, CPAP is no longer needed. Some patients have been able to stop CPAP, only to need it again months later.

Proper air pressure, face mask fit, and proper instructions on the use and care of the CPAP system coupled with support and encouragement from family members, the attending doctor, and the sleep center should help improve patient compliance.

State-of-the-Art Flow Generators to Treat Snoring/OSA

A newer form of therapy, known as Automatic Positive Airway Pressure (APAP) may provide additional comfort and therapy benefits for some patients, which will be discussed later alongside specific product features.

The choice of flow generator device can have a big impact on how well patients tolerate their therapy. There are several different kinds of devices available to serve a variety of patient needs. Patients who have difficulty adjusting to therapy may benefit from switching to a device that better suits their individual situation and preferences. For example, patients who travel a great deal may want a smaller, more convenient device. Patients who are losing weight may require different prescribed pressures over time, and there are appropriate devices designed for such patients. Additionally, some patients may simply find the pressure of positive airway pressure (PAP) therapy uncomfortable to breathe against, and there are devices designed to help those patients as well.

CPAP, APAP, and Bilevel

It is important for patients to be familiar with the different types of devices on the market so they can choose the best device for their needs. As mentioned before, CPAP devices deliver a constant pressure to splint the airway open during sleep. Another type of device is known as an Automatic Positive Airway Pressure (APAP) device. APAP devices use an algorithm to analyze the airway on every breath and automatically adjust the pressure so that the patient receives the lowest pressure necessary to keep the airway open. Another device is known as a Bilevel. Bilevel devices alternate between two different pressures. During inhalation, the pressure is higher in order to keep the airway open. When the patient exhales, a bilevel device drops pressure, making it easier for the patient to exhale.

The three types of devices have different benefits and are intended for different types of patients. The next few paragraphs describe the benefits and features of each type of device, and identify specific products that belong to each category.

CPAP Therapy—the Gold Standard

CPAP therapy is the gold standard for treatment of sleep apnea. The majority of patients who receive proper medical follow-up care are able to use CPAP comfortably and effectively. CPAP is the most commonly prescribed type of OSA therapy. CPAP devices are convenient, economical, and easy to use. The following devices include features that enable doctors and clinicians to access a patient's usage information using data cards, which helps patients by eliminating the need for expensive, time-consuming office visits. All of the listed devices are also available with optional humidification, which is an advantage for patients who experience side effects like congestion, sore throat, or nasal dryness from using CPAP.

APAP Therapy—For Patients With Changing Pressure Needs

APAP therapy was first introduced in 1999 and is considered the most significant improvement to OSA therapy in years. Sometimes referred to as "smart CPAP," APAP functions like a pacemaker for the upper airway. APAP devices continually adapt to a patient's changing pressure needs to deliver the lowest pressure necessary to maintain an open airway while ensuring maximum comfort and effectiveness. This automatic response is ideal for patients with fluctuating weight, changing fluid levels, seasonal allergies and varying medications, as well as patients who cannot tolerate CPAP. Patients who use APAP therapy often find it more comfortable and experience more benefits from their therapy, compared to CPAP.

Bilevel Therapy—For Patients Who Cannot Tolerate CPAP, or Patients With Coexisting Respiratory Disease

Bilevel devices are helpful for patients who need a lower pressure during exhalation. The lower pressure makes treatment more comfortable. Bilevel devices are also ideal for patients with other coexisting respiratory complications, such as restrictive or obstructive lung disease.

Improving Therapy

Getting the most benefit from therapy involves a combination of the right therapy, patient education, and setting realistic goals of use. Choosing the right flow generator, having a properly fitting mask, and using appropriate humidification to prevent and reduce side effects are very important to achieving success with sleep apnea therapy. Patients should consult their therapist with any questions (eg, how do I clean my mask?).

Knowing how to take proper care of therapy equipment is

also critical to ensuring therapy success. Patients must continue to ask questions if they are unsure of something even after getting home with the therapy. Most importantly, like achieving any goal, patients should set a plan for achieving the maximum level of device usage to ensure comfortable adjustment to the equipment. The standard goal for sleep apnea patients is to use it a minimum of four hours per night every night, but this may not be achievable the first week. Setting daily or weekly goals can help patients gradually work up to the target of four hours per night by the end of the third week.

Traveling with CPAP

Some patients worry that PAP treatment will interfere with their lifestyle or ability to travel. All of the PAP devices described in this book are fully portable and easy to travel with.

Air Travel

Some airlines have approved the use of PAP devices on long-haul aircraft. Before traveling, you should contact the airline to check whether any special requirements or restrictions apply. You should follow these recommended preparations.

Carry a letter from your doctor certifying your need for PAP treatment.

Obtain approval from the airline's Medical Services for use on the flight.

Have a copy of the approval letter from the airline.

Arrange seating close to a power source on the aircraft.

Confirm the type of power cord or adapter required by the aircraft.

On a recent trip back to the East Coast, I had no hassle carrying my APAP on the airplane as a second carry on. Security had no problem accepting the APAP as a medical device and it traveled through the X-ray machine safe and sound.

International Travel

Most PAP devices run on virtually any power supply in the world without the need for a power transformer. However, you will need a plug adapter appropriate for the country you are visiting. You can purchase plug adapters at electronics and travel stores.

Camping

If no AC power is available, a PAP device can operate with DC power and an appropriate inverter or converter. With the use of a suitable inverter or converter, a PAP device can operate from a battery supply (eg, in a truck or recreational vehicle). Some PAP systems may require a battery.

Local home medical equipment providers can assist patients in choosing a suitable inverter for their flow generator.

Patients should keep the following information with them while traveling:

Prescribed treatment pressure

Mask type and size

Home medical equipment provider's contact details

Sleep specialist's contact details

General practitioner's contact details

Health insurance information and documentation if possible.

Chapter 8

SURGICAL AND PHARMACOLOGICAL TREATMENT OPTIONS FOR OSA

Tracheostomy

Tracheostomy is rarely used anymore. It is used only in patients with severe, life-threatening OSA that do not respond to other surgical procedures or who cannot adapt to CPAP. In this procedure, a small hole is made in the trachea (windpipe) below the Adam's apple, and a tube is inserted into the opening. This tube stays closed during waking hours, while the patient breathes normally. It is opened for sleep so air flows directly into the lungs, bypassing any upper airway obstruction. Its major drawbacks are that it is a disfiguring procedure and the tracheostomy tube requires proper daily care to keep it clean.

Uvulopalatopharyngeoplasty (UPPP)

UPPP is a procedure used to remove excess tissue at the back of the throat (tonsils, adenoids, uvula, and part of the soft palate). This technique probably *helps only half of the patients who choose it.* It is rare, but possible, that negative effects can include nasal speech and regurgitation (back flow) of liquids into the nose during swallowing. UPPP is not considered as universally effective as tracheostomy, but does seem to stop snoring. It does not appear to prevent mortality from cardiovascular complications of severe OSA.

Although snoring is temporarily relieved in most cases, apnea may persist. The overall success rate of UPPP is reported to be about 40% (when success is defined as achieving an apnea-hypopnea index of less than 20). Therefore, it is very important to do a post-surgery sleep test to verify the success of the surgery and implement further treatment such as CPAP if necessary. It is difficult to predict which patients will benefit from this procedure and long-term side effects and benefits are unknown.

Nasal Surgery

Nasal surgery may be used alone or in conjunction with other procedures. However, alone it rarely cures the symptoms of OSA and snoring. Nasal surgery is useful in clearing the nasal airways of obstructions caused by polyps, cysts, or a deviated septum.

Laser-Assisted Uvulopalatoplasty (LAUP)

LAUP has received much attention recently as a treatment for snoring. However, its effectiveness in treating OSA has not been validated.

This procedure involves using a laser device to eliminate tissue in the back of the throat. This operation does not require general anesthesia or hospitalization as do more traditional operations of the upper airway. Like UPPP, LAUP may decrease or eliminate snoring, but it has not been reported therapeutic for OSA. Elimination of snoring without influencing OSA may carry the risk of delaying the diagnosis and possible treatment of OSA in patients who elect LAUP. *To identify possible underlying OSA, sleep studies are essential before LAUP should be performed.* The American Sleep Disorders Association's practice report on LAUP indicates that, "patients should be informed that the risks, benefits, and complications of LAUP have not been established."

Clinical symptoms alone are inadequate in ruling out OSA and may result in a failure to diagnose OSA. Pre-operative assessment must include a combination of clinical evaluation and an objective measure of respiration during sleep. A missed diagnosis could result in a patient undergoing an irreversible surgical procedure that does not address the true underlying disease pathology.

Maxillofacial Surgery

Genioglossal Advancement, Maxillary and Mandibular Advancement

These above surgeries are not yet widely available, although they appear to be promising in effectiveness in treating OSA. Genioglossal advancement enlarges the airway at the base of the tongue. This procedure may be combined with a UPPP. Maxillary and mandibular advancement enlarges the airway at the level of the soft palate as well as the base of the tongue. As with any surgery involving local or general anesthesia, there are greater risks associated with such treatments.

With any medical/surgical treatment for snoring or OSA, pre-operative and post-operative sleep studies should be conducted. The patient should understand fully the risks, benefits, and complications of any treatment that's under consideration. They should understand other alternatives such as CPAP and oral appliances, including the risks, benefits, success rate, and complications of these devices.

As mentioned earlier, after my sleep study I was examined by an otolaryngologist, ear, nose and throat (ENT) doctor, who explained that my loud snoring and mild OSA was due to an enlarged uvula and soft palate tissues in the throat area. These tissues were obstructing air flow during sleep. He said that surgical procedures reduce or eliminate OSA and snoring in some patients. He explained the risks, benefits, and complications of surgery, and I chose a non-surgical approach.

Recommend Exam by Board-Certified ENT with Good Track Record Treating OSA

After a sleep study has been conducted, I recommend

that those individuals who are loud, habitual snorers and those with OSA should consider an exam by a board-certified ENT specialist with a good track record in treating snoring and OSA patients. This examination should be done before deciding on a specific treatment for snoring or OSA.

The ENT can determine if the cause of apnea and snoring may be due to facial/skeletal deformities, deviated septum or soft tissue abnormalities in the nose or palate, tonsils or adenoids, all of which can be corrected.

It's advisable to know beyond a reasonable doubt that you truly need the surgery or procedure being prescribed. First, ascertain if the condition is a life-or-death situation. If it is not, then you may want to seek a second opinion, and maybe a third, if needed, to erase any doubt.

You will need to be armed with copies of all test reports including the doctor's analysis report relative to the tests and your examination. A breakdown of the facility's fees, doctor's fees, and all other fees associated with the procedure should be provided in writing.

You will need every bit of available information to assist you in making an intelligent decision on one procedure or another. You must have positive input from the facility and the doctor. Ask questions and make sure you get clear, specific answers from the facility and the doctor before making a decision to go ahead with surgery or any other procedure.

Most sleep disorders specialists agree that surgery is a treatment of last resort for snoring. Procedures that are reversible and non-invasive should be tried before surgery, even for OSA. Although physicians are not in total agreement on this statistic, the National Institute of Health, in its publication "Breathing Disorders During Sleep," states that surgery probably helps only about half of the OSA patients who choose it.

Surgical Reconstruction

Patients in whom OSA is due to deformities of the lower jaw may also benefit from surgical reconstruction. In addition, surgical procedures to treat morbid obesity are sometimes recommended for OSA patients.

Pre- and Post-treatment Management

The efficacy of a chosen treatment should be periodically verified. It is wise to perform a sleep study *before* and *after* they undergo surgical intervention. Once effective treatment has been initiated, all patients should be periodically re-evaluated for recurrence of symptoms, such as snoring and EDS, as well as cardiopulmonary complications. The primary care physician can play a key role in determining if patients are adhering to treatment and in monitoring conditions such as hypertension and coronary artery disease.

Hypertension treatment may need to be adjusted once OSA has improved. Patients who are adherent to treatment for OSA need positive reinforcement; those not adherent may require different treatment options. Patients who are on CPAP or other mechanical devices need to have their equipment evaluated periodically to ensure that the machine and mask are functioning properly. Oral appliances also need to be checked from time to time for proper functioning.

Pharmacological Treatments

No known medications are currently effective in the treatment of OSA. However, some physicians believe that mild cases of OSA respond to certain drugs that either stimulate breathing or suppress deep sleep. Acetazolamide has been used to treat central apnea, which is an absence of a signal from the brain which tells you to breathe. Tricyclic antidepressants inhibit deep sleep and REM, and are useful only in patients who have apneas during the REM state. However, REM sleep is important for both mental and physical good health and therefore tricyclics are not usually recommended for treating OSA.

"Medical management to reduce the size of the polyps," reports the Cleveland Mt. Sinai Center for Ear, Nose, Throat & Facial Surgery, "often requires a short series of steroid pills and nasal steroid sprays. Since the nasal steroid sprays have very little absorption into the blood stream, there are few, if any, side effects. Also, because the steroid pills are taken for a short time, they usually cause few side effects or few long-term problems."

Patients who suffer from hypothyroidism may also suffer snoring and obstructive sleep apnea as a consequence of their poor muscle tone. Thyroid replacement corrects the snoring and apnea. Therefore, ask your physician to test your thyroid function before he/she starts other treatments.

Oxygen administration sometimes benefits patients without producing any side effects. However, the role of oxygen in the treatment of sleep apnea is controversial; some experts think that it does not help, and it is difficult to predict which patients will respond to oxygen therapy.

Chapter 9

DENTAL OPTIONS TO TREAT SNORING AND OSA

Doctor Prescribed: Oral/Dental Appliances that Help Stop or Reduce Primary Snoring and Mild and Moderate OSA

In July of 1995, oral appliance therapy was first recommended by the American Academy of Sleep Medicine (AASM), formerly the American Sleep Disorders Association; for the treatment of primary snoring, mild to moderate obstructive sleep apnea syndrome (OSAS).

In 2006, the AASM released updated practice parameters for the treatment of snoring and OSAS with oral appliances. A summary of the 2006 updated practice parameters and some of the recommendations are listed on their Web site at www.aasmnet.org.

Oral or dental appliances may be an option for patients who snore and those with mild or moderate OSA. However, as with other treatments, they are not always effective for all patients. Appliances are used mainly for patients with primary snoring or with mild or moderate OSA, but do not suffer from severe OSA. There are various devices that displace the tongue forward or move the jaw to a forward position to improve breathing within the airway. Reported side effects of the devices include excessive salivation and minor joint discomfort. In addition, patients may experience changes in their bite. Only a dentist experienced in the uses of these devices should fit the patient with an appliance.

Sleep Study Required

A sleep study should be done before and after the appliance is fitted to evaluate the effectiveness. However, a follow-up study is not indicated for patients with primary snoring.

Oral appliance therapy is a sequential diagnostic process to maximize effectiveness of treatment while minimizing unneeded tests and costs. It is dependent upon effective communication between the patient, the attending physician/sleep specialist, and the dentist. This allows the patient to be involved in her therapy through understanding the diagnostic process, and permits her to make decisions for the immediate and long-term process. Throughout the therapy, the patients screen themselves out of or further into the diagnostic procedure.

The attending dentist begins by understanding the specific goals and objectives the patient wants to accomplish with the therapy. Is the oral appliance to serve as the primary treatment or as a secondary, substitute, or adjunctive treatment? Trial procedures are utilized to select an appliance type and customize its design to maximize comfort and clinical effectiveness. Continual feedback is required to effectively modify the trial appliances throughout this process. If the patient can benefit from a dental appliance, this process will help insure that the definitive appliance choice and design derived from trial procedures will be ideal for each patient.

Robert R. Rogers, DMD, is the founding president of the American Academy of Dental Sleep Medicine (AADSM), and has served as director at the Sleep Disorders Dental Society (SDDS) Resource Center and Chair of the SDDS Education and Curriculum Committee. The SDDS is now the AADSM.

"Various oral appliances have been shown to be effective in treating snoring and obstructive sleep apnea," says Dr.

Rogers. From the first oral appliance, which involved the repositioning of the lower jaw, developed by the French pediatrician, Pierre Robin, in 1934, to more recent innovations that hold the tongue forward, dentists have been actively involved in research and invention in their attempts to control airway obstructions and their consequences.

Dr. Rogers points out that a patient should only choose a dentist experienced in the field of dental sleep medicine in order to ensure a proper fit and adequate monitoring for the appliance's effectiveness. A sleep evaluation, ideally by a polysomnographic sleep study, should always be done prior to the construction of an oral device in order to distinguish whether the snoring is benign or a result of OSA. This involves the dentist and physician working together. If the patient does not respond favorably to behavioral treatments, such as weight loss and/or changing sleep position, or to devices such as CPAP, then dental appliances are an effective alternative. The most recent data support the role of oral appliances as first-line treatment for mild and moderate OSA.

Published dental reports indicate that the dental professionals present an untapped source of vital assistance treating persons at risk for serious sleep-related disorders, such as OSA and snoring, bruxism (grinding of the teeth), and temporal mandibular dysfunction (TMD), usually associated with pain syndrome or jaw stress. There are over 700 associated dentists who routinely perform these services throughout the United States as members of the AADSM. Web site: www.dentalsleepmed.org.

Most of the appliances used to treat snoring, and mild and moderate OSA are made of plastic, fitting over the teeth or tongue. According to Dr. Rogers, the small, mouth guard or retainer-like devices are easily adaptable and comfortable for most people. "They are also relatively inexpensive, non-invasive, and convenient as compared to other forms of treatment," says Dr. Rogers.

As stated before, the AASM published a policy statement in February 2006, outlining the guidelines for properly using oral appliances for the treatment of snoring and OSA. All dentists and physicians involved in this therapy should follow the practice parameters set forth by the AASM and AADSM.

Oral appliances may aggravate existing temporomandibular joint disease and may cause dental misalignment and discomforts that are unique to each device. Long-term follow-up care by a dentist is necessary to assess the development of any of these complications.

Types of Oral Appliances

There are many different types of oral appliances available. Selection of a specific appliance may appear somewhat overwhelming. Nearly all appliances fall into one or two categories. The diverse variety is simply a variation of a few major themes. Oral appliances can be classified by mode of action or design variation.

TRD - tongue retaining device

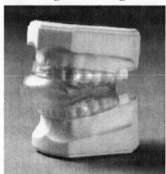

Photography provided by AADSM formerly Sleep Disoder Dental Society. All rights reserved.

Tongue Retaining Appliances

Tongue retaining appliances function by holding the tongue in a forward position by means of a suction bulb. When the tongue is in a forward position, it serves to keep the back of the tongue from collapsing during sleep and obstructing the airway in the throat.

Mandibular Retaining Appliances

Mandibular Repositioning Appliances function to reposition and maintain the lower jaw (mandible) in a protruded position during sleep. This serves to open the airway by indirectly pulling the tongue forward, stimulating activity of the muscles in the tongue and making it more rigid.

It also holds the lower jaw and other structures in a stable position to prevent opening of the mouth.

SNOR.X

The SNOR.X device was invented by R. Michael Alvarez, DDS, a dentist, board-certified in sleep disordered breathing by The American Academy of Dental Sleep Medicine, also certified in Oral Systemic Balance Therapeutic Systems located in Fremont, California.

MRD - mandibular retaining device

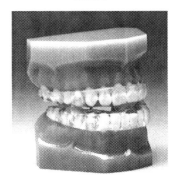

Photography provided by AADSM formerly Sleep Disoder Dental Society. All rights reserved.

This device was invented with the permission of Dr. Charles Samelson, MD, to act as a trial device before a customized TRD (Tongue Retaining Device) would be prescribed and constructed. This device is generic and can fit almost anyone. The simple design and instructions for use are the highlights of this device.

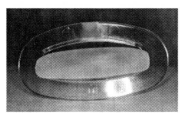

Front View

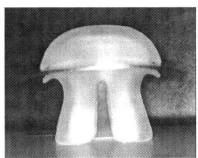

Bottom View

New Oral Systematic Balance Therapy

The road to physiologic balance can be reached with the use of the Oral Systemic Balance Therapy. This therapy allows the tongue the freedom to be positioned in an ideal area. The pioneering work of Farrand C. Robson, DDS, has revealed to us a variety of neuromuscular reflexes and therapies that impact a multitude of daytime symptoms that commonly occur in our patients. Not only the people with sleep disorders suffer, but so do their friends and family that are with them whether it is during the day or night.

The tongue is now, not captured in a bulb but guided by physiologic contact with an oral device. The device appears to be variations of mandibular advancement appliances and TMD splints. There is a patented system built into these new Oral Systemic Balance Devices which is unique in therapy for OSA, UARS, TMD, and fibromyalgia.

Unraveling the Mystery of "TMJ"

Many people are confused about all the initials and names that refer to temporomandibular joint (TMJ) disorders. This article is to discuss the various terms, what they mean and why this jaw joint disorder, or dysfunction, has become known so many different ways including:

TMJ—"T" stands for the temporal bone of the skull. "M" stands for the mandible or condyle. "J" stands for joint which connects your lower jaw to your skull.

TMD—Temporomandibular Disorders

Craniofacial Pain—head and facial muscle disorders

CMD—Craniomandibular Disorders, which are head and jaw disorders

MPD—Myofascial Pain Dysfunction Syndrome

"Myo" is the Greek word for muscle and "fascial" refers to connective tissue in muscle.

All these terms refer to problems involving both the jaw joints and muscles of the head, neck, and face. Unfortunately,

"TMJ" is the term the public learned years ago when the disorder was actually recognized. We all have two TMJs, one on each side of the head in front of the ears. So, when someone says, "I have TMJ," it's true from the standpoint that we all have two. In actuality, the correct term when a patient suffers with TMD symptoms means they have a TM joint Dysfunction. Many TMD dentists have also termed the problem as CMD or MPD which are all accurate terms. Because the public learned to express their problem using "TMJ," even though it is incorrect, it is hard to change years later.

The TM joints are the two joints that connect the jaw to the skull. They are located on each side of the head in front of the ears. When they are displaced, they cause mild discomfort to severe pain involving the head, neck, and face. It is estimated that as many as one in every four Americans (mostly women between the ages of 25 – 40) suffer from one or more of these signs that indicate a TM disorder:

Headaches

Earaches, stuffiness or ringing ears

Pain behind the eyes

Click, pop, or grating sound in the jaw joints

Limited mouth opening

Unexplained tooth pain

Dizziness for no known reason

Locking jaws

Neck pain or stiffness

Difficulty swallowing

Less common symptoms of shoulder stiffness, fingers, and back pain can also be signals of a problem. Even snoring can be an indication of TMD which James Mosley has discussed thoroughly in this book. In fact, most TMD sufferers also have a snoring or sleep apnea disorder.

Treatment

Most often, a TMD dentist is the main provider of diagnoses and treatment. He may work in conjunction with physical therapists, chiropractors, or massage therapists in the best interest of the patient. It is important to find a dentist who is qualified, trained, and experienced. This means s/he has a deep interest and dedication to treating head, neck, and facial pain patients. Because there are no mandatory courses in dental school for the dentist to learn how to treat TMD or sleep disorders, a dentist must choose to learn. He must take continuing education courses at his own expense and time. This is why it is important to find a dentist who has acquired the special training necessary to properly treat these disorders. Treatment of TMD consists of the patient wearing an orthotic (splint) over their teeth for a period of time. Sometimes, depending on each individual case, the orthotic only needs to be worn at night to prevent clenching and grinding to help relax the muscles. Other times, it is necessary to wear the orthotic 24 hours a day for a few months until the pain or spasm has dissipated.

The dentist goals for TMD treatment is first to deal with pain and muscle spasm, and second to restore jaw function and stabilization of the correct joint position. Usually, an oral appliance (orthotic or splint) is initially the suggested mode of treatment.

The goal for treating sleep disorders is to dilate or open the airway by altering the position of the lower jaw to treat snoring or mild to moderate OSA. In more serious sleep apnea situations, a sleep appliance can be an adjunct to other treatments such as CPAP and surgery.

This article on "Unraveling the Mystery of TMJ" was written by Sharon Carr who is a TMD sufferer herself and understands what others go through when enduring such a disorder. She has been a frequent guest on TV and radio to alert and educate the public about TMD. As founder of TMData Resources in Albuquerque, her purpose is two-fold:

- To offer help for TMD sufferers through education.
- To work with dentists and other health-care professionals for practice development and marketing consulting.

Proper Choosing of a Physician and Dentist for Diagnosis/Device Fitting

Arthur M. Strauss, DDS, is a co-founder of American Academy of Dental Sleep Medicine (AADSM) and a noted practitioner in dental management of sleep disorders. He estimates that 90% of dentists making oral appliances are not proficient, or even experienced in applying the TRD and MRD, and that over 80% of these have no experience with TRDs. Furthermore, fewer than 10% of dentists ordering oral appliances from dental laboratories and distributors are members of the AADSM. He also stresses that most physicians or sleep disorders specialists are unfamiliar with the protocol and trial procedures recommended by the AADSM, namely that treatment should be relevant to the patient and trial procedures are designed to wed the patient with an appropriate appliance.

Initially, the AADSM defined trial procedures as testing with both TRD and MRD type appliances to determine which basic "type" is appropriate before narrowing the selection down to the specific design of the "type" (TRD or MRD). Now the AADSM has been non-specific in its description of trial procedures. Strauss feels that this is "not" consumer oriented, but oriented to a paucity of members trained in TRD use and streamlining treatment to a factory conveyer belt approach over a science based one. This has resulted in "trial procedures" where practitioners not testing with trial appliances but essentially going directly to a definitive MRD design chosen on clinical judgments based upon examination alone. If the MRD is not effective or not tolerated by the patient, a few members familiar with and competent in use of the TRD will then test the patient with one. Strauss claims that credentialing criteria for becoming a Diplomate of the AADSM does not necessitate demonstrating proficiency or even familiarity in the use of the TRD oral appliance.

A new approach to oral appliance therapy, developed by Farand C. Robson, DDS, called Oral Systemic Balance® (OSB) Therapeutic Systems focuses on restoration of impaired oral function that primarily impacts speaking, swallowing, and breathing. OSB based on the work of Robson has revealed a variety of neuromuscular reflexes and therapies that impact a multitude of daytime symptoms that commonly occur in patients. This sophisticated approach to care, through modification (tweaking) of size and contour of the space housing the tongue alters tongue posture, position, and both proprioceptive input and output of the tongue. Adding or removing less than 0.25 mm thickness to the contour of teeth or the appliance covering teeth or tissue will alter tongue posture, speech, and breathing. With this, one can see secondary changes in pulse oximetry, patient posture, and heart rate variability. Determining where to make the modifications and how much modification is needed separates this from the "crude" approaches the dental profession has been using. OSB requires extensive practice and training. Robson updates practitioners personally to enable them to hone their skills continually, especially their communication (observing, listening, and questioning) skills required to appropriately adjust the appliances for maximizing their positive effect.

Beware of Unscrupulous Practitioners

In Dr. Strauss' opinion, when the media limits its report to specific appliances rather than treatment as a therapy with a protocol. It trivializes the concept of oral appliances and appropriate procedures associated with them. To minimize the likelihood of choosing under-trained or unscrupulous practitioners, Dr. Strauss offers the following suggestions:

1. Seek education on these issues.
2. Try to find a sleep specialist, board-certified by the Ameri-

can Board of Sleep Medicine for diagnosis and treatment recommendations. Their work is purely diagnostic, so they are less apt to be prejudiced toward certain treatments.

3. Ask if the sleep specialist works with dentists utilizing multiple appliances, especially the two basic types (TRDs and MRDs) which are consistently used in trial procedures for appliance selection. Ask how much experience the dentist has had in this field. Also explain that you would like to hear that the dentist has completed at least a few dozen cases or credible explanation supporting his or her experience.

4. Get verification by asking the dental office to explain what types of appliances they work with and what specific designs they most often use. Then ask them to describe their treatment protocol. If they do not include both TRDs and MRDs and trial procedures as originally defined by the AADSM you should continue searching for one who does. If you find a dentist also certified in Oral Systemic Balance® Therapeutic Systems, you have most likely struck it rich!

Chapter 10

ORAL SYSTEMIC BALANCE® THERAPEUTIC SYSTEMS: A NEW THERAPEUTIC APPROACH

Oral Systemic Balance® Therapeutic Systems provides a new, noninvasive therapy that is based on major scientific advances resulting in a better understanding of how the body mechanisms keep the airway open and the consequences of this system breaking down.

Snoring and Obstructive Sleep Apnea (OSA) are the result of a breakdown in the body's ability to keep the airway in the throat open. When this occurs, the tongue is able to fall back into the throat (pharynx) and either obstruct or partially obstruct the air passage which can result in snoring, OSA or a multitude of other concerns. How the tongue maintains its position in the mouth so that it does not go back into the throat is critical.

These new findings reveal more about the normal protective mechanisms of the body keeping the throat airway open so that we can easily breathe, swallow and speak. The recruitment of this biologic system by Oral Systemic Balance® therapies allows snoring and OSA to be managed along with a wide variety of other symptoms including "TMJ" and many other pain conditions and agitation states. This new knowledge and therapy is the result of the work of Doctor Farrand C. Robson and is now available through certified Oral Systemic Balance® (OSB) practitioners.

This system uses oral devices that have some similarities

with the dental orthotics that have been used in the treatment of snoring and OSA, however OSB therapy is quite different in that they do not solely rely on alteration of jaw position to keep the tongue from falling back into the throat. OSB Therapies address snoring and sleep apnea at the level of their origin. In doing so it also impacts other symptoms associated with the underlying system problems. Oral Systemic Balance Therapies applies new knowledge of the effect that the shapes and contours of the teeth and other oral structure have on the tongue and throat airway. In this way, snoring and OSA are better managed as breathing, swallowing, and speaking are made easier.

The magnitude of the impact of this therapy on the body can be understood when we realize that keeping the throat open is the most important body function. The physiological changes that occur as breathing, swallowing and speaking are restored are so significant that a unique and specialized evaluation and monitoring process is needed to manage the treatment and allow each person greater awareness of their symptoms and a more active role in their care.

The throat is kept open by a variety of body compensations. The most basic of these is the underlying tightness or tone of the tongue muscle when we are fully relaxed which determines how the tongue sits in the mouth, as well as the throat. There must be enough tension in tongue muscle to hold the tongue forward so that it does not fall back and block the throat airway when we are relaxed. This has important implications in the cause of snoring, OSA, and other conditions. This has not been understood prior to Doctor Robson's work.

The modification of this muscle tone with Doctor Robson's patented orthotics allows greater ease of the primary oral functions such as swallowing, speaking, and breathing. OSB Therapy directly alters this muscle tone by the tongue's contact with the teeth and other structures in the mouth. This management of the muscle activity in the tongue muscle has direct application to the treatment of snoring and OSA.

OSB Introduces Daytime Therapy

Day time therapy is part of OSB Orthotic Therapies since maintenance of an open throat is not just a night issue, even though treatment of OSA and related symptoms has up until now been focused on nighttime concerns. There are many serious day symptoms associated with snoring and OSA. If there is obstruction of the throat when we relax at night, it is to be expected that day time problems will also exist. The structure and form of the throat are present 24 hours a day, we are just not able to adapt to these problems at night as well as we do in the day. Specially designed unobtrusive day time orthotics have had marked benefit for many OSA and other sleep disordered breathing patients.

Clinical Results Of OSB Therapy In Snoring And Obstructive Sleep Apnea

Doctor Roy Hakala, a certified OSB practitioner in St. Paul Minnesota, provided OSB Therapy for a surgeon who was so severely affected by snoring and OSA that he was falling asleep during surgery! CPAP use actually made his condition worse and his sleep clinic referred him for OSB Therapy including an OSB oral sleep orthotic. The surgeon summed up his results of OSB Therapy in the simple phrase, "This has changed my life!"

Another example of success is from Doctor John D. Walsh, a certified OSB practitioner in Anchorage, Alaska who provided OSB Therapy for a local physician, Doctor Sandra Denton. She has stopped snoring and reports that she "noticed a number of health benefits immediately." Doctor Denton states, "I am thrilled with the results of the Robson OSB appliance and have encouraged many of my patients to get it. One 78-year-old patient no longer requires her CPAP machine, which she had been using for two years. She also no longer snores."

Richard Simpson of Rialto, California also experienced beneficial effects as he shares, "A desire to eliminate sleep apnea brought me to Doctor Robson. Upon starting to wear a dental device I felt that my tiredness was gone. . .overnight that twenty year old pain from a right knee injury was gone. . .also gone were the pains in my lower back and under my left shoulder blade. . .I've regained that three-quarters of an inch in height that I had lost." Even greater for Richard, "Mornings, I awake feeling refreshed and able to accomplish something worthwhile, which wasn't the case before. I'm really feeling great!" Anyone who has, or is close to someone who suffers with snoring problems can appreciate these remarks.

Introduction To A New Science

Oral Systemic Balance® Therapy is innovative and scientific and developed from over twenty-five years of work by Doctor Farrand Robson of Tacoma, Washington. OSB Therapy helps people with snoring, sleep disordered breathing, muscular pain problems, and other concerns by recruiting normal body mechanisms that restore or maintain normal function.

All the air you breathe goes over the back of the tongue and through the throat. Any disturbance in the normal muscle reflex mechanisms that maintains muscle tone and tongue position will result in some level of interference with the primary oral functions of breathing, swallowing, and speaking. Many of these muscular reflexes that keep the throat open are the result of the shape and position of teeth and are modified by routine dental procedures. When the tongue is properly positioned and airflow is unrestricted, oral functions are effortless and effective and sleep is restful and pleasant.

Difficulty with breathing, swallowing, and speaking often can be traced to the configuration of the mouth. This is most often related to problems involving muscle tone of the tongue.

An excessively narrow or broad mouth, crowded teeth, loss of teeth, bulky dentures or partial dentures, and other oral conditions all can interfere with tongue space as well as interfere with the normal reflex mechanisms that maintain muscle tone. In such cases, the only place the tongue can go during oral function is backward, into the throat. Lack of appropriate tongue space can be apparent when observing the tongue, and is obvious when the tongue is scalloped or when tongue thrust is present.

Disordered breathing is usually caused by tongue obstructing airflow down the throat. In this situation, every inhalation requires extra effort and puts negative pressure (suction) on the soft tissues of the throat. The chest wall works harder than normal to draw air in, and the resultant forceful and turbulent airflow over these enlarged tissues produces snoring. The continued effort of the chest wall that is required to maintain breathing interferes with normal cardiovascular dynamics and interrupts and/or prevents deeper and more restful sleep stages. People who snore often sleep lightly or fitfully, awakening at the smallest disturbance, and often blaming their awakenings on the need to empty the bladder. They still feel tired on rising and often can sleep for ten or more hours without feeling fully rested.

There are several systems that aid in the body's adjustment to keep the throat open. One of these compensations is clenching and grinding of the teeth which causes a reflex called the Jaw Tongue Reflex (JTR) that actually opens the throat more and makes breathing easier. This is a frequent cause of Jaw pain and headache pain in the temples and behind the eyes. When severe, many people can have nausea and be very sensitive to light and sounds.

Forward head posture, which changes the posture of the whole body, is another compensation that lets us breathe more easily. Like the clenching of teeth, forward head posture may be associated with muscular pain as muscle contracts to maintain breathing. The weight of the head in a forward position puts an enormous strain on the body, especially muscles of the neck, shoulders, and back. This can result in pain anywhere in the axial skeleton. People with this posture may experience difficulty and have less stability with Physical Therapy and Chiropractic care since restoration of normal head posture makes it more difficult to breathe freely. The head and body will again move forward to reopen the throat. OSB Therapy can reduce or eliminate the need of these posture alterations and allow the body to self correct. In this way, OSB Therapy complements these other therapies.

Another major compensation that the body makes for an obstructed throat is to activate the sympathetic "fight or flight" component of the Autonomic Nervous System (ANS), releasing neurotransmitters such as adrenaline. Adrenaline facilitates muscle function, allowing stronger and more rapid muscle contraction, which helps the body adjust to maintain an open throat. This is the reason that we feel more on edge at the same time we are experiencing muscular pain. Adrenaline also raises the heart rate, which is one reason people with nighttime breathing problems, also known as choking, may wake with the heart racing. There are many other effects from this adrenaline release, including digestive and stomach acid concerns.

The adrenaline that is needed to maintain breathing is often associated with diagnoses of anxiety, depression, and even panic attacks. As Doctor Robson of OSB frequently says, "My patients who are 'viciously choking' appear to be anxious, depressed, and on edge." The on edge feelings are often thought to be "stress," "anxiety," or other psychological concerns but in reality are a survival "fight or flight" response.

The OSB Therapeutic Systems Approach

Oral Systemic Balance® Therapy is a process that occurs

over time and starts with a specific diagnosis. A comprehensive history, as well as a highly specialized interview process, physical examination, radiographs (x-rays), pulse oximetry, heart rate variability testing (HRV), postural analysis, and diagnostic dental casts are combined with the patient's own account of their chief complaints and health concerns. Treatment is designed to establish a more open throat that allows for greater ease of swallowing, speaking, and breathing. Once the ease of these primary oral functions has been established, the sympathetic nervous system no longer needs the fight-or-flight reaction. The patient often feels safer and more relaxed than they remember ever being.

HRV is a measure of the level of physiologic function and adaptability that quantifies the activity of the sympathetic and parasympathetic nervous systems. It is a predictor of cardiovascular disease and stroke. The National Heart, Lung and Blood Institute has acknowledged the increased risk of stroke

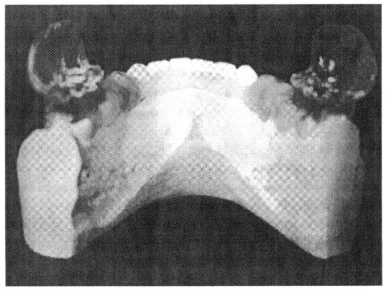

One of several orthotic designs available through OSB laboratories.

for patients with jaw related muscle pain (TMJ) problems and sleep disordered breathing (SDB). Use of HRV provides a special level of safety for the patients, especially those with multiple systemic disorders.

The OSB treatment system uses intra oral orthotics, patented devices that look a little like orthodontic retainers and that fit comfortably over the teeth, usually the lower teeth. The OSB laboratory individually designs and fabricates the orthotics. Shapes and forms are built into and added onto these orthotics that trigger reflex changes in the tone of the tongue so that the tongue has a place to rest in the mouth and prevents the tongue from falling back into the throat. The jaw is held at the most appropriate vertical and horizontal dimensions to support ease of the primary oral functions. Once a patient takes a few easy, deep breaths with a fully adjusted orthotic, head posture improves, healthy and vital facial skin tones appear, head and neck pain fades and leaves, and the patient is free to enjoy the relaxed and peaceful, whole-body effects of effortless breathing.

Follow-up radiographs are taken to be sure that the OSB orthotic is providing optimal improvement in jaw position, tongue posture and opening of the throat.

A variety of OSB orthotic designs are available to allow for individualized treatment. Some of the orthotics prescribed fit on the lower and/or upper teeth, whereas others fit both upper and lower teeth at the same time and have either a rigid or a mechanical connection between the upper and lower components. Orthotics designed for daytime wear are inconspicuous and often enhance the clarity and tone of the voice. Many patients with snoring or OSA will require separate nighttime orthotics, like the one pictured, that stabilize the jaw and tongue position dependably during sleep.

Many people have difficulty tolerating standard dental appliances that do not support the reflex patterns to maintain

Same Day Analysis of
Before and After Intitial Treatment With An OSB Orthotic

Cayden initially had head and neck pain, sleep disturbance, chest tightness, and agitation feelings. These symptoms all resolved with initial OSB Therapy. "I can breathe now. I just feel so much better!" This is what Cayden Luce of Tacoma, Washington said after receiving OSB Therapy.

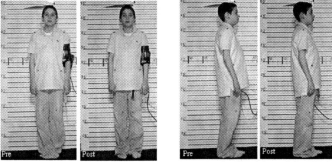

These posture analysis photos were taken on the first day of Cayden's treatment. Notice his 1-inch height increase!

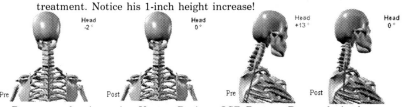

Posture evaluation using VenturaDesigns OSB Posture Pro analysis shows Cayden's initial head tilt 2 degrees to the left and forward 13 degrees. Initial posture breakdown was needed for Cayden to be able to breathe.

Cayden's father, Dan Luce has this to say about his son's OSB Therapy: "His resting oxygen saturation was dangerously low and his resting heart rate rather high. After being fitted with an initial OSB dental orthotic to assist his breathing, his resting heart rate and oxygen saturation percentages nearly inverted. His pale skin immediately turned a healthier pink color. I am unable to find words to adequately express my joy at having been introduced to Doctor Robson's practice and the weekly opportunity to be among his most amazing staff."

appropriate muscle tone. Some appliances can be bulky and can steal space from the tongue. Such appliances can actually increase nighttime clenching and aggravate morning headaches, cause Temporomandibular Joint (TMJ) pain, and excessive salivation. OSB appliances do just the opposite: They

provide appropriate tongue space and provide normal neuromuscular reflexes that support normal muscle tone. This results in decreased clenching and improved breathing.

Doctor Arthur Strauss, an OSB practitioner in Falls Church,
Virginia, treated Reverend Dan Horner who said, "It has occurred to me that the mandibular repositioning devices
(MRDs) are so crude and stress inducing in comparison (to
OSB orthotics). They (other MRD) held my lower jaw in an
unnatural position and filled my mouth with plastic. The OSB
nighttime appliance is so comfortable in comparison. I feel
relaxed when I am wearing it and my jaw is no longer sore
like it was after a night wearing an MRD."

Patient Participation In Treatment

The OSB interactive interview and diagnostic testing allows the patient to understand the source of their symptoms
so that they actively can participate in their care and know
that they can be well. When a patient is finally able to relax
and experience the feeling of well being, they become aware
of what it feels like to breathe, swallow, and speak more freely.
Once this occurs, they can assess the benefit of any orthotic
and actively participate in their treatment. They no longer
have to maintain the same intense behaviors that they had
previously needed to maintain adequate ease of breathing,
swallowing and speaking.

What Is Being Said About OSB Therapy

"This therapeutic approach is nothing short of an historic
medical breakthrough," says Doctor Rusty McDougal, a certified OSB practitioner, following the provision of OSB care for
a number of his patients.

Virginia Stull of Dayton, Ohio was a long-time sufferer of
multiple symptoms before she saw Doctor Richard Quinttus,
a certified OSB practitioner. Now Virginia exclaims, "My
memory has improved and I am no longer lethargic. I no
longer have severe lower limb muscle spasms and hand cramp-

ing." She also reports that her need to get up at night has gone from three to six events to not more than once a night. In a testimonial she writes, "You are making a difference in people's lives. You most definitely have in mine."

After receiving treatment from OSB certified practitioner, Doctor Gordon D. Wagoner of Flora, Indiana, Nancy S. Cripe wrote, "I can honestly say that as long as I wear my OSB (orthotic) every night, I am totally pain free. I cannot remember the last time I took anything for pain. Previous to that day (of receiving the orthotic), I took Advil on a daily basis. I sleep much better at night and wake up feeling more rested, I do not snore, and rarely have a headache."

Doctor Stephen Levine of Kentfield, California, CEO and president of Allergy Research Group, wrote in a letter to Doctor Robson, "Its only been four days since I last visited with you and significant changes have taken place. I noticed an increase in stability in terms of a steady energy the very first day I wore the appliance. And on Friday I took my dogs for a run and noticed a considerable difference in my exercise tolerance, without real effort. Since adulthood I have managed myself with exercise, meditation and careful diet but I was aware of some autonomic imbalance. So now for the first time, in a very long time, I experience a sense of physical stability that is new. Thank you for your fine work."

E.J.O. from the Southeastern USA who saw Doctor Robson for OSB therapies shares his experience with on edge feelings: "My search for release from defensive, judgmental, abrasive internal dialogue and behavior and from physical feelings of tension, stress and anxiety has spanned the past 40 or so years. . . I had driven away most friends, living somewhat in isolation, and was feeling what seemed to be the footprints of advancing time. After a series of adjustments I find myself with a feeling of great peace, no more need to fight, deep love and compassion, a sense of coming home. It is now safe to live at home in this body and be in the world. After all else had failed, this works."

After receiving OSB Therapy from a certified OSB practitioner, Doctor John Laughlin III, of Ellsworth, Wisconsin, Deb shared, "The biggest changes occurred when the OSB appliance was inserted. The first night I was taking a lot of deep breaths, my husband noticed, it was a big change for me to not be snoring, and restless. Now I'm able to breathe and get fresh air. The 'brain fog' has lifted. I'm able to do a lot more things. I'm a student, and studying is so much easier. The sun is brighter. I now have hope."

Doctor Michael Alvarez of Freemont, California, a certified OSB practitioner, treated Liz Leslie with OSB Therapy and she said, "The (OSB) oral appliance I have been sleeping with works!!! I had a normal sleep study with the appliance in my mouth."

Doctor Arta Vakhshoori of San Jose, California, a certified OSB practitioner, notes the dramatic improvement she has seen in her patients since providing this therapy. One of her patients in particular was diagnosed with OSA and was unable to tolerate CPAP. The first evening this patient received OSB Therapy he slept for twelve hours straight for several days in a row. He now uses the orthotics and not the CPAP.

After watching a relative suffer for over two years with diagnosed Restless Leg Syndrome (RLS), sleeping an average of only two to four hours a night, and fifty pounds overweight, Doctor Randle H. Egbert of Milford, Ohio, a certified OSB practitioner, provided intensive OSB Therapy utilizing several orthotics. Now his relative has significantly decreased symptoms of RLS, is sleeping longer periods, "seems alive again" and "has energy, mental sharpness, and most of all smiles again."

Doctor Thomas Layman of Richomond, Virginia, a certified OSB practitioner, also witnessed profound results for Butch

Bolden when he treated him with OSB Therapy. After suffering for over thirty-five years with OSA, sinus headaches and fear of choking to death, Butch saw dramatic changes when he started treatment. Six weeks into treatment he reports that the snoring is gone, his "fight for life has ceased," he awakes rested, started dreaming again, awakens with no sinus stuffiness or headaches, and many other improvements.

Doctor Vince Sessions of Kirbyville, Texas, a certified OSB practitioner shares his thoughts on OSB Therapies, "I have never seen such well documented and in depth information on the tongue and oropharynx. I have encouraged my colleagues to look into the OSB course, and will continue to encourage other dentists and physicians, for this valuable training." Doctor Leonard Kundelof Stamford, Connecticut, also a certified OSB practitioner, agrees with Doctor Sessions and adds, "OSB breaks down the negativity until nothing is left but peace and silence. In my own practice, it allowed me to help people to get out of their negative loops and move on with their lives."

Doctor Robert J. Rowen heard about the life-changing results that were occurring with OSB therapies and made a point of personally and critically evaluating these reports. He recounted his first visit to Doctor Robson's office, where his best friend, Ronald MacDonald had been suffering for over thirty years from OSA. Doctor Rowen shares that, when Ron received his orthotic, "Instantly, (Ron) became more relaxed, his blood-oxygen saturation jumped five points to normal, and he exclaimed, 'I can breathe!'" Additional information regarding Dr. Rowen's evaluation of OSB Therapy can be read in previous issues of Second Opinion Newsletter at www.secondopinionnewsletter.com.

Doctor Brian J. Smith of Eureka, California, also an OSB practitioner expressed the feelings of many when he wrote, "Doctor Robson, I can't thank you enough for developing this

therapy to improve overall health."
Is It For Me?

Although evaluation by an OSB-certified dentist is needed
to determine if any specific person is a candidate for this
therapy, most people suffering with snoring or other sleep-
related disorders and chronic head and neck pain problems
will benefit from OSB therapy. One quick self-test involves
body posture: If it is easier for you to breathe (swallowing
and speaking may also be noticed) when you slouch, letting
your head drift forward, than when you are standing tall like a
soldier with your back to a wall, you will probably benefit from
OSB therapy.
Extraordinary Results

The OSB diagnostic and therapeutic system was developed by Doctor Farrand C. Robson over twenty-five years of
dedicated work. He evaluated jaw dysfunction and jaw related
pain conditions in order to more fully understand the relationships between the jaw, teeth, throat, and the rest of the body
and establish the origin of these conditions. The primary focus of Doctor Robson's work is to provide a systematic therapeutic system that can be broadly used by other practitioners
to benefit the millions of people who suffer with these problems. OSB currently trains doctors around the country in
this therapy and updates them on the continuing scientific
and technologic advances generated by Doctor Robson.

Doctor Wayne Whitley of Fredericksburg, Virginia, a certified OSB doctor, stated that, "The innovative and original work
of Doctor Farrand Robson of Oral Systemic Balance® has connected the dots for those suffering with these and related
maladies and the healthcare providers seeking to assist them
in their journey. My health has been optimized and I can now
optimize the health of those that seek care at my office."

Doctor Robson explains the extraordinary results that
doctors and patients are seeing with OSB therapies as "the

closer we are to the cause of a problem, the better and more rapid are the results of treatment." Treating the cause, instead of just the symptoms, and partnering with other practitioners including chiropractors, optometrists, neurologists, psychiatrists, and others produces profound results. Specialists are continually impressed by the way their treatment results are enhanced by OSB therapy that addresses the underlying anatomical conditions. It has always seemed unlikely that the broad list of symptoms many patients have would be the result of several independent disorders, all striking a single person at one time. OSB diagnosis helps get to the root cause of many of these disorders and OSB therapy helps resolve a whole spectrum of symptoms at once.

Doctor A. Joseph Williams III of Nashua, New Hampshire, a certified OSB doctor, states, "I now recommend this therapy to everyone I can. I have witnessed remarkable results in everyone I have treated."

Contact Information For Patients And Doctors

Patients who want to locate a licensed OSB dentist or want more information on OSB Therapy may call 1-800-977-1945.

Doctors can become certified as OSB practitioners after a series of courses and upon meeting specific educational and practical requirements. Those interested in receiving OSB training may call 1- 800-977-1945 for additional information.

Chapter 11

WHERE TO GET HELP AND GUIDELINES ON SELECTING PHYSICIANS AND SLEEP CENTERS

The National Commission on Sleep Disorders Research, in its eight public hearings nationwide, heard witness after witness describing the devastating impact of sleep disorders and sleep deprivation. One curious observation they made was that patients do not often complain about, and doctors do not investigate, sleep habits. The Commission estimates that this affects the lives of approximately 50 million individuals "whose lives could be improved or saved..."

The Commission says that "undiagnosed or mistreated sleep disorders are a common experience of sleep disordered patients. Up to 10 million Americans stop breathing in their sleep." The findings report that *about 95% remain undiagnosed*, although these patients often seek doctors' advice about the symptoms commonly associated with sleep disorders (headaches, high blood pressure, depression, low energy).

These startling conclusions spell out that the person requiring medical attention these days must become his or her own self-made "expert," becoming fully knowledgeable about the condition requiring medical attention and having full understanding of the treatment options available.

This person must become savvy regarding sleep disorders centers, the types of physicians involved, the testing they perform and available treatments (which could include surgery or non-invasive procedures), not to mention the cost of every aspect of this process. Most of us do more research when we buy a car or a television set than when we choose a doctor or a hospital. There is no consumer magazine that rates doctors and hospitals the way *Consumer Reports* rates air conditioners. Undoubtedly our bodies and overall well-being deserve more attention than these machines.

It would be hard to rate physicians, sleep centers, and sleep disorders specialists in the way a consumer rates appliances, but when providers are willing to give you an abundance of information, it's a good sign. It shows that they are responsive to patients and confident of their capabilities.

The World Wide Web

The Internet is a good source to get information about doctors, dentists, hospitals, and sleep centers. Countless Web sites provide detailed information on health-care professionals, their facilities, credentials, speciality, performance, policies, and practices.

Securing as much information as you can is the key to choosing the correct professional and sleep center for your needs. You are starting on the right path by reading a book designed to provide you vital information on these subjects. There are also a number of organizations whose goal is to provide information, education, and support to sleep disordered individuals and their families.

Where To Get Help

The names of those organizations and their addresses, telephone numbers, and Web sites are listed as follows:

American Academy of Dental Sleep Medicine (AADSM)
One Westbrook Corporate Center, Suite 920
Westchester, IL 60154
(708) 273-9366 Fax: (708) 492-0943
www.dentalsleepmed.org

American Academy of Otolaryngology
Head & Neck Surgery Foundation
One Prince Street
Alexandria, VA 22314-3357
(703) 836-4444 Fax: (703) 684-4288
www.entnet.org

American Academy of Sleep Medicine (AASM)
Formerly the American Sleep Disorders Association
One Westbrook Corporate Center, Suite 920
Westchester, IL 60154
(708) 492-0930 Fax: (708) 492-0943
www.aasmnet.org

American Board of Sleep Medicine
One Westbrook Corporate Center, Suite 920
Westchester, Il 60154
(708)-492-1290 Fax: (708)-492-0943
www.absm.org

The American Sleep Apnea Association and A.W.A.K.E.
Support Group
(Alert, Well And Keeping Energetic) Network
1424 K Street NW, Suite 302
Washington, D.C. 20005
(202) 293-3650 Fax: (202) 293-3656
www.sleepapnea.org

Joint Commission on Accreditation of Healthcare
Organizations
One Renaissance Boulevard
Oakbrook Terrace, IL 60181
(630) 792-5000 Fax: (630) 792-5005
www.JCAHO.org

Medical-Dental Education Network
2188 Peralta Boulevard, Suite D
Fremont, CA 94536-3941
Fax: (510) 713-6794

Narcolepsy Network, Inc.
P.O. Box 294
Pleasantville, NY 10570
(401) 667-2523 Fax: (401) 633-6567
www.narcolepsynetwork.org

National Center on Sleep Disorders Research
6701 Rockledge Drive Suite 10042
Bethesda, MD 20892
(301) 435-0199 Fax: (301) 480-3557
www.nhlbi.nih.gov/sleep

National Heart, Lung and Blood Institute (NHLBI)
6701 Rockledge Drive Suite 10042
Bethesda, MD 20892
(301) 435-0199 Fax: (301) 480-3557
www.NHLBI-NIH.gov

National Institute of Child Health & Human
Development
P.O. Box 3006
Rockville, MD 20847
(800)-370-2943
www.nichd.nih.gov

The National Sleep Foundation
1522 K Street N.W. Suite 500
Washington, D.C. 20005
(202) 347-3471 Fax: (202) 347-3472
www.sleepfoundation.org

Oral Systemic Balance
1901 South Union Avenue
Suite B5010
Tacoma, Washington 98405
(800) 977-1945
www.oralsystemicbalance.com

Restless Legs Syndrome Foundation
819 2ⁿᵈ Street, SW, P.O. Box 7050
Rochester, MN 55902
(507) 287-6465 Fax: (507) 287-6312
www.rls.org

TMData Resources
800 Branding Iron S.E.
Albuquerque, NM 87123
(800) 533-5121 Fax: (505) 332-1661
www.tmdataresources.com

If you require surgery and you wish to know whether the hospital or ambulatory care center you are considering is accredited by the Joint Commission on Accreditation of Healthcare Organizations, you need to contact the Joint Commission Center at (630) 792-5000.

Readers in Scotland, Northern England; Southern England, Wales or Northern Ireland should visit *http://www.sleepmatters.org/* to locate a sleep clinic in your area. Readers in other countries should visit... *www.ersnet.org/ers/default.aspx?id_fiche=229474 to locate a sleep clinic in your area.*

National Organization Dedicated to Sleep Apnea Awareness
The American Sleep Apnea Association (ASAA) is a na-

tional voluntary health agency dedicated to individuals with sleep apnea and their families.

ASAA was founded in 1990 as a nonprofit organization by persons with apnea, along with concerned health-care providers and researchers. The ASAA's mission is simple:

The ASAA is dedicated to reducing injury, disability, and death from sleep apnea and to enhancing the well-being of those affected by this common disorder. The ASAA promotes education and awareness, research and continuous improvement of care.

Patient and Family Members Support Group

The ASAA A.W.A.K.E. Network plays a crucial role in the ASAA's efforts to educate the public and to serve as an advocate for those affected by sleep apnea. "A.W.A.K.E." is an acronym for "Alert, Well, And Keeping Energetic," characteristics that are uncommon in persons with untreated apnea. The A.W.A.K.E. Network was founded in 1988, as a mutual self-help support group for persons affected by sleep apnea. The ASAA A.W.A.K.E. Network is now composed of more than 250 groups in 45 states. A.W.A.K.E. meetings are held regularly, often with guest speakers. Topics may include advice on complying with CPAP therapy, legal issues affecting those with sleep apnea, weight loss, current trends in such fields as oral appliances, and new research findings.

In other efforts to fulfill its mission, the ASAA publishes the bimonthly newsletter, *Wake-Up Call* which provides useful, accurate, and objective medical information, as well as (in light of their patient advocacy role) articles on health, wellness, research news, and social and legal issues facing people with sleep apnea.

ASAA's 1996 president, renowned researcher, and sleep disorders specialist, Dr. Kingman P. Strohl, is a professor of medicine at Case Western Reserve University in Cleveland, OH.

Dr. Strohl's interest has focused on the management and

consequences of sleep apnea. He was one of the first researchers to identify that obstructive sleep apnea can run in families. Dr. Strohl has always been and continues to be a strong patient advocate. **The World's Greatest Book states, "As iron sharpens iron, so one man sharpens another."** I have found the A.W.A.K.E. meetings very interesting and a valuable source for information on OSA, its pitfalls, treatments and follow-up health care.

Networking with people who have experienced similar sleep problems, or who have a common interest in wellness, can be very valuable, especially since the paramount objective should be to gain as much knowledge as possible about the sleep problem, the diagnosis process, and the best available treatments.

By interacting with others who share this diagnosis, the sense of isolation common to sleep apnea patients can be alleviated. In addition, the educational benefits of such a group provide patients with a better understanding of the medical nature of their disorder, helping them to be more responsible for their own health.

The A.W.A.K.E. program provides a beneficial experience for the health-care providers and the patients. Health-care providers benefit from the feedback from the patients and the opportunity of increased involvement in the patient follow-up from hospital/sleep center to home. This encourages better communication between the patient, the hospital staff, and the home health-care company.

A.W.A.K.E. meetings are open to those who believe that they may have a sleep problem, as well as patients, their mates, family members, and friends. To locate the A.W.A.K.E. group in your area, contact The American Sleep Apnea Association and A.W.A.K.E. Support Group Network. The address, telephone number, and Web site are listed previously in this chapter.

Health Care Highlights
Managing Your Own Personal Health Care, Health-care Services and Health-care Plan

Some health-care plans have specific exclusions for sleep testing or for certain diagnoses like sleep apnea, narcolepsy, insomnia, and other sleep disorders. Be sure that your health-care plan will cover all or most of the expenses of an evaluation by a sleep specialist who is certified by the ABSM. Board-certified sleep specialists are highly trained in sleep medicine to provide the best possible consultation, testing, diagnosis, and to recommend treatment for all sleep disorders.

If your current health-care plan will not cover the services of a board-certified sleep specialist, then you may want to consider changing to a health-care plan that will cover all or most of the costs. Individuals who suspect that they may have a sleep problem and those who have a sleep problem should become responsible managers of their own health care, investigate their health-care services, and examine their health-care plan.

As previously mentioned, untreated sleep apnea is a serious life-threatening disorder that can result in death. Further, those who have OSA and drive a vehicle are at a higher risk of a fall-asleep crash. Whether your health-care plan covers the services you require is certainly an issue to overcome; however, the greater issue is: *Do you choose life or death?* You may need to make a sacrifice; it may come down to foregoing a vacation, or maybe having the family car repaired, rather than purchasing a new one. The money you save could go toward getting your sleep problem repaired and possibly saving your life.

Once you have been properly tested and treated, your activities should be more enjoyable, with the peace of mind in knowing that you have taken responsible steps to get your sleep problem corrected. Also your family members can enjoy life much, much more, knowing that you made a wise decision to get your sleep problem treated first.

The good news is that once OSA has been treated, the chances of having a fall-asleep crash are also reduced and the chances of living a healthier, longer life are greatly increased.

Choosing a Sleep Disorders Center/Hospital

Before selecting any facility, you should ask these questions:

1. *Is a preliminary evaluation conducted for the type of diagnostic services that will be needed?*

Two tests can be used to diagnose sleep apnea, and other sleep disorders: the *polysomnography* and the *multiple sleep latency test.* Doctors continue to try to develop other simple and economic procedures for the early diagnosis of sleep apnea, but to date these two tests are the most definitive.

Polysomnography is a group of tests that monitors a variety of functions during sleep. These include electrical activity of the brain, eye movement, and muscle activity for sleep stage assessment, heart rate, respiratory effort, airflow, blood oxygen and/or carbon dioxide levels for respiratory and cardiac assessment and leg muscle activity for period limb movement assessment. Other tests may be ordered depending on a particular patient's needs. Polysomnography helps to distinguish between different sleep disorders, sleep apnea, periodic limb movements, bruxism, sleep seizures, etc. These tests are used to diagnose sleep apnea and to determine its severity, as well as assess or rule out other sleep disorders.

The Multiple Sleep Latency Test is done during normal working hours. It consists of observations, repeated every two hours, of the time taken to reach various stages of sleep. In this test, people without sleep apnea, narcolepsy, etc., take more than 10 minutes to fall asleep. On the other hand, patients with sleep apnea or narcolepsy fall asleep fairly rapidly. When it takes the patient an average of less than five minutes to fall asleep, it is considered severe pathological sleepiness. If it takes between five and ten minutes to fall asleep, then they have moderate pathological sleepiness. This test is important because it measures the degree of objective excessive daytime sleepiness and also helps to rule out narcolepsy, which is associated with the increase of REM sleep (dream sleep) during naps.

Pulmonary function tests are not diagnostic for sleep apnea patients, but may show coexisting lung disease. To make a definitive diagnosis of sleep apnea, the doctor should order an all-night evaluation of the patient's sleep, breathing, and other vital functions related to sleep.

2. *If high-tech equipment, such as polysomnography, is used in procedures, are staff members properly trained to use and care for the equipment?*

Technicians are a key part of the sleep disorders center. A Registered Polysomnography Technologist ® (Psg. T.) has been tested and certified in all technical aspects of sleep evaluations by the Association of Polysomnographic Technologists. Most good sleep disorders centers typically have at least one experienced sleep technician, usually a Psg. T., who is the chief technician and one or more other technicians. The technicians prepare patients for the sleep test, attaching various sensors on the body to monitor and record brain waves, eye movements, muscle tone, heart rhythm, breathing and breathing effort, as well as oxygen in the blood. This enables the accurate identification and determination of the severity of breathing problems as well as other problems that can disturb sleep.

Some other considerations in selecting the proper facility are:

1. *Does the facility have a written description of its services and fees?*

2. *Is the organization able to help you find financial as-*

sistance if you need it?

3. *Will your insurance company reimburse you for the cost of the procedure? If so, at what percentage?*

4. *What is the facility's success record for the specific procedure you need?*

5. *Does the organization explain the patient's rights and responsibilities?*

Choosing the Right Doctor for Your Needs

The following are some questions that should be asked when choosing a doctor.

1. *What are the doctor's credentials?*

Board certification or an international equivalent is a sign that doctors are highly trained in their field. Doctors who specialize should be board certified in the specialty in which they are practicing. Most specialists have a national board which is responsible for setting the standards doctors must meet in order to be certified. Doctors who are board certified in their specialty have completed the amount of training that the specialty board requires, and have practiced for a specified number of years in that specialty and have passed a difficult examination in their specialty area. Some excellent doctors are not board certified. Board certification, however, is generally a good indication of competence and experience.

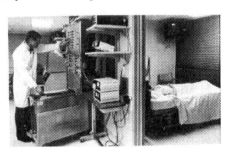

2. *What is the specific training of the doctor who will be performing the evaluation?*

A true sleep specialist is board certified by the American Board of Sleep Medicine (ABSM). They are MD's or PhD's who have undergone intense special training and are certified by examination to evaluate and interpret sleep tests, diagnose, and recommend appropriate treatment for all sleep disorders. Sleep specialists are directors of a sleep disorders center that have the appropriate staff and equipment to monitor and record sleep and diagnose sleep disorders. The sleep specialists communicate the results and their recommendations to you and your family physician. If you do not have a family physician, the sleep specialist, or one of the center's medical associates can implement treatment.

3. *Does the doctor have a written description of his/her services and fees?*

4. *Does the doctor provide you with information detailing the procedure and possible risks?*

5. *Does the doctor conduct a sleep study before offering surgery as an alternative? And is a post-treatment sleep study prescribed?*

6. *Are the physician and staff receptive to your questions?*

7. *How much experience does the doctor have?*
It may be important to ask whether the doctor performs all procedures at one medical center/hospital or at several. If the doctor performs procedures at more than one medical center or hospital, this increases the volume, but could mean the doctor is working with different teams. The teams, therefore, might not have as much experience working together as they would if the doctor was working with the same team at the same hospital all the time.

8. *What is the doctor's success rate for the procedure prescribed?*
Choosing a doctor or sleep disorders center/hospital is often influenced by values. You may want to go to a facility that is close to home. You may want a hospital with a specific religious affiliation. But when you need specialized medical care for a sleep disorder, it is essential that you also include in your decision a doctor who is board certified by the ABSM. These doctors may have a private center or have a center at a hospital. These qualify indicators will help you determine the

best facility and doctor for treatment.

The Role of the Home Health-care Company

Home health-care companies, also known as durable medical equipment companies, provide medical equipment and supplies to hospitals and other medical facilities, as well as to patients at home. Some full-service home health-care companies include field respiratory therapists who visit the OSA patient at home, setting up the CPAP system as ordered by the doctor, as well as providing instructions and follow-up on the device's use and maintenance. Some sleep disorders centers also provide CPAP equipment to sleep apnea patients.

Diagnostic Sleep Studies Conducted in the Home

Some full-service home health-care companies specialize in helping physicians, clinics, and hospitals obtain sleep studies of their patients with sleep disorders.

Using the newest non-invasive technology, these companies provide sleep testing in the patient's home. These tests focus on the detection and treatments of sleep disorders. However, some of the home health-care companies may not be supervised by a board-certified sleep expert; therefore, the types of tests and the recording quality may not be as advanced as testing in a sleep center, resulting in a misleading or wrong diagnosis.

Home health-care companies typically offer in-home sleep studies for patients who have difficulty with hospital-based overnight testing. Patients in nursing homes and in intensive care units who cannot be moved need the tests brought to them. Persons who have difficulty in traveling, people in smaller communities where there are no sleep center programs, insomnia sufferers requiring multi-day testing, those needing follow-up care treatment for OSA, sufferers of alveolar hypoventilation syndrome, nocturnal myoclonus, restless legs syndrome, or another diagnosed sleep disorder, and children under 12 are all persons who may benefit from sleep studies conducted in the home.

Some sleep disorders centers are able to perform sleep tests in the home, but typically prefer the sleep laboratory testing for better quality and control.

Help for Veterans at VA Centers

Most full-service Veterans Administration Medical Centers are able to diagnose and treat sleep apnea and other sleep disorders. Non-service-connected veterans are screened to determine their eligibility when applying for treatment. According to the Department of Veterans Affairs pamphlet, "Health Insurance Carriers, VA & You—The Non-service-Connected Veteran," the veteran will be asked questions regarding his/her health-care insurance coverage. The pamphlet does state, however, "Eligibility for VA medical care is not affected by your insurance coverage. Your eligibility is based, in part, on your financial status and the availability of particular services at your local VA medical facility."

I have found in my own experience at my local VA Medical Center that the quality of the sleep specialists are of the highest caliber. This is probably due to the fact that some of the specialists are also on the staffs of other highly reputable hospitals in the community at large.

New Generation of Computerized Sleep Disorders Centers Now Being Implemented

Awhile ago I underwent an overnight sleep study at a sophisticated computerized sleep disorders center. My previous two sleep studies were monitored by a polysomnography machine. The main reason for the latter sleep study was to verify the air pressure on my CPAP system to determine if it was still adequate.

The sleep technician who attended me indicated that the computerized system has been in place for about three months, and the system offered some new enhanced features. He mentioned features, such as the ability to perform more critical tests, faster collection of data, faster sorting and out-putting of data, and hard-drive disk storage capability.

The technician indicated that it would take about a year to fully evaluate the new computerized system.

I saw the old polysomnography machine (large in size) sitting in the observation room still connected but abandoned, giving way to the new wave of sophisticated medical technology, the computerized sleep disorders center.

Chapter 12

CHRONIC SLEEP DEPRIVATION AND FATIGUE IN AMERICA: IT TAKES A SIESTA

Causes of Sleepiness

The following is an excerpt from the National Commission on Sleep Disorders Research report, "Wake Up America: A National Sleep Alert":

Each human being requires a specific amount of sleep in each 24-hour period to maintain optimal waking function. If an individual obtains less than this optimal dose, he will be less alert the following day. Moreover, sleep loss accumulates from one night to the next as a "sleep debt." Therefore, sleep of durations that represent only a modest loss of sleep on a single night may produce a serious sleep debt when sustained over several nights. The more sleep lost each day, the greater the sleep debt and the larger the impairment.

In the laboratory, sleep debt can be measured by assessing increased sleep tendency, negative mood, and performance decrements. In the real world, the consequences include learning impairments, discord in interpersonal relationships, errors and accidents. Because individuals often do not recognize that they are sleepy, they seldom guard against inappropriate sleep episodes. Much like the intoxicated driver, sleepy drivers do not realize they are incapable of adequate performance and may deny drowsiness and impairment. When the individual does acknowledge sleepiness, it is often attributed mistakenly to boredom, to an overly warm environment, or to a heavy meal; rarely is drowsiness linked to the true cause—the quality and quantity of prior sleep. Sleepiness also may result from medication, alcohol consumption, or age-related deterioration of sleep found in the elderly.

America's massive sleep debt results from a complex interplay of technological advances, needs that compete with sleep, widespread ignorance, and to the ubiquitous disorders of sleep.

Voluntary Chronic Sleep Deprivation

Over the past 100 to 125 years, we have reduced our average nightly total sleep time by over 20%. Yet, no available scientific evidence suggests that we have developed a reduced need for sleep or that our ancestors slept too much. The change in our sleep behavior has paralleled technological change in our society. While our ancestors had few choices of activity for the evening hours, we can now choose from a wide variety of activities. The invention of electricity has enabled much activity to continue past sunset—now, 24-hour operations are commonplace.

A convincing body of scientific evidence leads the Commission to the conclusion that many Americans are sleep-deprived and, therefore, are sleepy during the day. Surveys of children's and adolescents' sleep habits conducted in 1910-1911 found that eight- to twelve-year-old children averaged about 10.5 hours of sleep per night; 13- to 17-year-old adolescents averaged 9.5 hours. A 1968 survey found that the average number of hours of sleep experienced by each group had declined by 1.5 hours. *It is assumed that the appropriate amount of sleep is the amount that will allow the individual to awaken voluntarily, without the use of an alarm or other environmental influences.* When allowed to sleep without environmental influences for 14 consecutive days, young adults, who report typical nightly sleep durations of 7.5 hours, have been shown to average 8.6 hours per day.

Diminished Productivity and Impaired Performance

Over 30 years of laboratory research document the influence of sleep loss on human functioning. Sleepy individuals are less ambitious and less productive. Sleep loss impairs performance on cognitive tasks involving memory, learning, logical reasoning, arithmetic calculations, pattern recognition, complex verbal processing, and decision-making. For example, reduction of sleep time to five hours a night for only two nights significantly reduces physiological levels of alertness, impairs vigilance, and worsens arithmetic ability and creative thinking. Loss of as little as three hours of sleep in a single night can slow human reaction time significantly, a change which can be dangerous in situations such as driving.

The consequences of reduced sleep time—whether caused by sleep disorders, voluntary sleep deprivation, or circadian factors—include diminished mental and physical health, increased mortality, lowered productivity, and increased incidence of errors and accidents.

Increased Morbidity and Mortality

The Commission found that habitual short sleepers are at risk of increased morbidity and mortality. According to several studies, individuals who report sleeping six hours or less a night experienced poorer health than those sleeping seven to eight hours a night. Moreover, a nine-year follow-up study found that individuals sleeping fewer than six hours each night had a 70% higher mortality rate in comparison to those who slept seven or eight a night. This association remains significant even after controlling for age, gender, race, physical health, smoking history, physical inactivity, alcohol consumption, and social support.

The Commission found abundant information suggesting that the relatively short habitual sleep duration associated with shift work significantly increases the risk of morbidity and mortality. Shift workers suffer a higher incidence of ill-

ness than non-shift workers, including gastrointestinal and
cardiovascular disorders. Although the psychosocial consequences of sleep loss and shift work have received little scientific attention, the toll is likely to be great. Sleep deprivation is known to result in a more negative mood. For example,
a recent study reduced the nightly sleep of adolescents by
two hours for five consecutive nights, from the usual 8 to 9.5
hours to 6 to 7.5 hours. At the end of just five nights of restricted sleep, the study group showed significant increases
in dysphoria, feelings of poor health, and unhappiness. Prior
research involving longer periods of sleep restriction indicates
that the negative mood swings may persist for weeks or
months.

Night workers and rotating shift workers have a three- to
five-fold increase in psychosocial problems, such as an inability to find time for family obligations, community service, or
other routine activities. Shift work has enormous social consequences that are exacerbated by the emotional vulnerabil-
ity associated with reduced sleep time. The Congressional
Office of Technology Assessment has documented marital
problems and community alienation as just two of the results
of the strain imposed by work schedules.

Few Americans appear to know the facts that are most
important.

1. Sleep loss is cumulative.

2. The sleep debt and chronic sleep deprivation are cam-
ouflaged by endogenous and exogenous stimulation and circadian rhythm effects. Thus, an individual may not feel sleepy
at one time of the day, but may experience the sudden onset
of completely disabling drowsiness when all stimulating influences are withdrawn. This is what happened to the third mate
on the bridge of the Exxon *Valdez* a few minutes after midnight on the night of the grounding, as well as countless drivers at about the same time of the day.

3. Adolescents appear to need as much sleep as younger children and perhaps more and, thus, the marked reduction of time in bed that occurs during adolescence has profound and far-reaching consequences.

4. Napping can immediately relieve dangerous drowsiness. The Commission found that the mission of society is seriously undermined by chronic sleep deprivation and fatigue. Knowing the facts of sleep and sleep deprivation can only help our citizens foster the growth of a safe and productive society.

More Sleep—Jim's Radical Approach to Help Overcome America's Massive Sleep Deprivation Problem

I recommend a goal of nine hours sleep per day to help overcome the huge chronic sleep deprivation problem in America! Especially for those individuals who work in industries that require shift-work, fast reaction, and/or quick strategic decisions.

The thought that one can go without sleep is dead wrong. Many in our society view operating on minimal sleep day after day as a sign of being mentally and physically tough, as if depriving oneself of sleep is proof of superior abilities.

However, researchers are clearly pointing out that our normal efficiency, alertness, and creativity are challenged at even the normally recommended eight hours of sleep a day. Eight hours of sleep a day is viewed by sleep experts as acceptable; however, some people can operate on less than eight hours of sleep per day, but nine hours of sleep per day appears to be the optimal amount of sleep for maximum body and mind efficiency.

Most Americans operate on less than eight hours sleep per day. Researchers indicate that in 1950 the average American slept eight hours per day, but in 1996, the average is seven hours sleep per day. Researchers also say that many individuals require more than eight hours sleep per day to operate at their best.

The brain is the part of the body that needs sleep. The "frontal lobe" is the part of the brain that is used in figuring out math problems, negotiating turns, making judgment calls, planning, initiating behavior, or sustaining behavior along with situations that require decision-making and fast reaction.

The National Commission on Sleep Disorders Research reported that in two different studies when subjects, whose typical nightly sleep duration was 7.5 hours, were allowed to sleep without influences such as an alarm or other environmental influences, they averaged 8.9 hours sleep per night, nearly 1.5 hours more each night. These studies support the fact that our sleep needs remain constant throughout adulthood. Most of us still require the same amount of sleep that we did when we were younger, and will continue to do so even into the golden years.

As mentioned before, there is no available scientific data to suggest that we have developed a reduced need for sleep or that our ancestors slept too much. The change in our sleep behavior has paralleled technological change in our society. Some of the compelling factors that influence sleep deprivation are: demanding work schedules that include 10 to 16 hours of work per day, shift work, and time spent commuting to and from work. Some individuals work two or three jobs each day, which usually results in a reduction of available sleep time.

Social and family demands also play their part in robbing individuals of sleep. In addition, environmental influences, such as street and highway noise generated by trucks and cars, along with airplane and railroad noise all contribute to fragmented sleep, which can result in sleep deprivation.

Studies show that individuals who are sleep deprived become much slower, clumsier, more forgetful, more easily stressed, and generally suffer from lower mental alertness. These individuals may actually fall asleep at inappropriate times, which may put the individual and others at risk for accidents and death.

Stress is considered by most sleep researchers to be the Number 1 cause of short-term sleep deprivation. Some major factors that trigger stress are death of a spouse or family member, marital problems, job-related pressures, and personal injury or illness.

The good news is that usually the sleep problem disappears when the stressful situation passes.

The following Stress Factor Table (on the next page) is not an exact scientific measurement or analysis. It is meant to visually portray a concept and allow you to think about how you handle stress.

Changes in our lives are certain to cause stress. Knowing that some of life's events are more stressful than others and trying to anticipate and plan for such changes may help us. The Social Readjustment Rating Scale helps us consider such changes.

When stress levels are decreased, the potential of becoming sleep deprived also decreases.

How to Determine if You Are Sleep Deprived!

According to sleep researchers, one simple rule-of-thumb to determine if you are sleep deprived is to try and take a nap early in the afternoon. If you fall asleep right away (less than five minutes), chances are that you are sleep deprived. Conversely, if you cannot fall asleep or it takes 10 minutes or more to get to sleep, then you have probably had adequate sleep.

For some individuals, a second question may need to be answered. Do you sleep excessively during the weekends? If the answer is yes, you have probably built up a sleep debt during the week, thereby leaving you sleep deprived.

Most importantly, the third consideration should be to ensure that you do not suffer with a sleep disorder.

Snore No More!

STRESS FACTOR TABLE

Life Events	Mean Value
1 Death of spouse	100
2 Divorce	73
3 Marital separation	65
4 Jail term	63
5 Death of a close family member	63
6 Personal injury or illness	53
7 Marriage	50
8 Fired at work	47
9 Marital reconciliation	45
10 Retirement	45
11 Change in health of a family member	44
12 Pregnancy	40
13 Sex difficulties	39
14 Gain a new family member	39
15 Business readjustment	39
16 Change in financial state	38
17 Death of a close friend	37
18 Change to a different line of work	36
19 Change in number of arguments with spouse	35
20 Mortgage or loan over $10,000	31
21 Foreclosure of mortgage or loan	30
22 Change in responsibilities at work	29
23 Son or daughter leaving home	29
24 Trouble with in-laws	29
25 Outstanding personal achievement	28
26 Wife begins or stops working	26
27 Begin or end school	26
28 Change in living conditions	25
29 Revision of personal habits	24
30 Trouble with boss	23
31 Change in work hours or conditions	20
32 Change in residence	20
33 Change in schools	20
34 Change in recreation	19
35 Change in church activities	19
36 Change in social activities	18
37 Mortgage or loan less than $10,000	17
38 Change in sleeping habits	16
39 Change in number of family get-togethers	15
40 Change in eating habits	15
41 Vacation	13
42 Christmas	12
43 Minor violations of the law	11

Priority Goal for Those Who Are Sleep Deprived

I encourage those who are sleep deprived to strive to get nine hours of sleep a day in order to get the best optimal mind and body performance, plus maintain some reserve, which we can all use every day, even if we aren't sleep deprived.

In his book *Sleep Thieves*, Stanley Coren says, "Perhaps it is time for policymakers, health workers and all the rest of us to wake up. The data is now quite clear that sleepiness, the direct result of not enough sleep, is a health hazard to individuals. It also may be a danger to the general public because of the possibility that a sleepy individual might trigger a catastrophic accident such as those associated with Chernobyl, the Exxon *Valdez* and the space shuttle *Challenger*."

Thus, researchers have shown us that the concept our society holds that those who (are free of sleep disorders, but) sleep 9 or 10 hours a day are "sleepy heads," or lazy, may be incorrect thinking in most cases. In fact, they may be wiser than the rest of us. Sleep researchers indicate that the best solution to overcome sleep deprivation is to get adequate amounts of sleep.

Daily Naps Can Help Prevent Sleep Deprivation

To achieve the nine hours of sleep per day goal, one may sleep nine hours continuously each night (not always the perfect solution), or 8 to 8.5 hours at night and a one-half or one-hour nap in the afternoon. The idea of an afternoon nap, such as the siesta, is common practice in other cultures.

The mid-afternoon slump most of us experience, even when we've slept well, suggests that the human body may be meant to nap. A regular afternoon siesta isn't likely to become a part of North American culture, but an occasional restorative nap may be a very good idea, particularly if you need to tap into an alertness reserve and a longer period of sleep isn't an option.

There's increasing evidence that a fifteen- to twenty-minute nap can improve alertness, sharpen memory, and generally reduce the symptoms of fatigue. If you're coping with the impact of lost sleep from last night or you know you're going to lose sleep tonight, a nap can help you through. In fact, it could be the difference between life and death if you're planning on a long drive with less than your regular quotient of sleep.

FAA Proposes 10 Hours Rest to Help Overcome Sleep Deprivation

The Federal Aviation Administration (FAA) has proposed a rule that would increase from 8 hours to 10 hours the minimum rest time for crew members between commercial flights. This rule was proposed in December 1995, after pilots raised the issue.

The author believes that similar guidelines should be established for air traffic controllers, truck, bus, and train drivers.

CONCLUSIONS

Author Recommends That Physicians Screen All New Patients for Sleep Disorders. Family Members and Friends Must Become Proactive

Some time ago I ran into an acquaintance of mine, Mike. A 41-year-old owner of a retail establishment, Mike is a big man, mild-mannered, and patient with his customers.

In our conversation, I discovered that Mike had recently undergone a triple bypass heart operation. His surgery was successful and his recovery progressing nicely. Mike had quit smoking, dropped his fast food and cola habit, reduced his TV-watching time, and increased his walking and exercise regimen.

What caught my attention was Mike's comment that he had suffered from a severe breathing problem while he was in the recovery room following his bypass. He was startled awake when he felt the doctor inserting a breathing tube down his throat. The doctor at that time stated he suspected Mike had OSA. At that point, Mike told the doctor he had been using a sleep machine to help him breathe at night. The doctor was speechless to discover *after* the surgery that Mike had a breathing disorder.

Mike could have suffocated to death in that recovery room—not from the bypass surgery, but from OSA due to an incomplete medical history. The doctors, nurses, and others had asked Mike endless questions about his health; however, they failed to ask any sleep-related questions, although Mike had all the symptoms associated with OSA. He was overweight, had smoked, did little or no exercise, had high blood pressure, an uncontrolled diet, a size 17½ inch neck, and was an extremely loud snorer with bouts of EDS.

In addition to Mike's profile, Mike's father was also a very loud snorer. All of these factors are key indicators that put individuals at risk for OSA, but the doctors didn't ask any questions related to sleep before performing major heart surgery on Mike.

Had Mike died while in the recovery room, the cause of his death possibly would have been linked to complications resulting from the heart surgery, and not to the actual cause, suffocation due to OSA.

In years past, how many others have died senseless post-surgery deaths, simply because the medical professionals failed to ask vital questions about sleep in the gathering of patients' medical histories?

Mike is a blessed man, but I suspect that there have been many people not so blessed, and they didn't live to tell the true story.

A curious thing, Mike mentioned that his father died at the age of 57, from a heart attack. However, Mike was sure his father died from suffocation due to OSA.

Challenge to Health-care Professionals

I strongly recommend that upon the initial patient visit, all doctors, including dentists—in fact, all medical professionals—should ask the patient to complete a standard set of sleep-related questions designed to uncover OSA and other major sleep disorders.

Also, patients must become proactive in their own health care. Thus, if the doctor does not ask questions related to sleep, the patient should inform the doctor of any sleep problems or concerns which will be helpful in treating the whole person.

The National Commission on Sleep Disorders Research reported that the most important barometer of awareness of sleep disorders and sleep deprivation is at the level of primary care clinical practice. When experiencing illness, most patients first will go to their primary care physician. For the majority of those suffering from sleep disorders, proper identification at this point can lead to early appropriate treatment. Some of the most prevalent serious sleep disorders are among the most straightforward to identify. For example, when an overweight, heavily snoring, middle-aged male with a neck size 17½ complains of excessive fatigue, it is highly likely that he has treatable obstructive sleep apnea.

According to a 1991 Gallup Poll, physicians failed to diagnose, or even identify, *one in three adults* who suffers from insomnia. Most narcoleptics contact as many as five physicians before attaining a proper diagnosis; 15 years may be spent between symptom onset and diagnosis. The excessive cost of mis-diagnosis and inappropriate tests and treatment were highlighted by many Commission witnesses. Once properly diagnosed, a good percentage of those with sleep disorders can be treated. Clearly, identification of sleep disorders at primary care level may reduce the cost of medical care for millions of patients. In addition, the author believes that proper diagnosis at the primary care level could help to save countless Americans lives.

Challenge to Health-care and Sleep Associations

I recommend that the American Medical Association, American Academy of Sleep Medicine, The American Sleep Apnea Association, and the American Academy of Dental Sleep Medicine work together to develop and implement a standard set of sleep-related questions which all doctors and dentists can use to detect those who are predisposed to OSA and other major sleep disorders.

A questionnaire similar to the one outlined in Chapter Five of this book could be designed for patients' use.

Challenge to Mate, Family Members, Friends, Room-mates and Coworkers to Become Proactive.

As stated before, most people who snore and have OSA do not know the extent of their snoring, and they do not know that they have OSA. Therefore the author has designated the mates, family members, friends, roommates and coworkers of a person who snores loudly as the Snorers First Line Responders (SFLR). Sleep apnea is a life-threatening disease when left untreated, therefore the SFLR can in fact save a life.

The SFLR are empowered to help their loved one or friend by completing the SFLR Quiz and the Snoring Assessment Study outlined in Chapter Five. I challenge the mates, family members, friends, roommates, and coworkers to become proactive and help their loved ones or friends to live longer and healthier.

There is a saying, where there is smoke, there is fire. I say, where there is loud snoring, there may be obstruction in the throat/nasal airway and a strong possibility there is sleep apnea. And like fire, sleep apnea can and does take lives. I encourage you not to play Russian Roulette with your life. Instead, if you are a chronic snorer, see your primary care physician without delay; it could mean the difference between life and death. As for me, I chose treatment and life.

Challenge to Researchers

I would applaud the researcher who develops a more user-friendly method to treat moderate to severe OSA. Moreover, I am sure that millions of sleep apnea patients would be elated if researchers could find a cure for OSA.

Challenge to the Transportation Industry

I recommend that the transportation industry implement sleep deprivation and sleep apnea awareness programs. These programs should be designed to educate the management force and its employee base on the effects of sleep deprivation, fatigue, and sleep disorders in the workplace, especially those driving trucks, buses, trains, and aircrafts or airplanes.

Implementation of these awareness programs could greatly benefit the commercial trucking, airlines, busing, and railroad industries by saving countless lives and millions, perhaps billions, of dollars in liability. The NCSDR report has revealed that, "In an objective, all-night sleep study of 159 truck drivers, 46 percent had moderate to severe obstructive sleep apnea, a syndrome known to increase the risk of accidents due to falling asleep." The report also stated that, "Sleep-related motor vehicle accidents cause hundreds of thousands of accidents, claim the lives of over 10,000 Americans annually, and cost society more than $30 billion per annum."

In the transportation field, the consequences of drowsiness can be especially serious, because of the dangerous or valuable cargo carried and the traveling speeds of trains, airplanes, trucks, and buses. The consequences may be all the more serious when an accident occurs near a heavily populated site or a fragile ecosystem.

Also, sleep researchers indicate that sleep deprivation can slow a person's response time to stimuli, and it can cause a lack of concentration and short-term memory deficits. Hence, airline and military pilots, air traffic controllers, truck, bus, and train drivers can be especially vulnerable to the effects of sleeplessness. This is due mainly to the sedentary nature of their jobs, which is further compounded by rigorous schedules that put them at higher risk of work-related errors and accidents.

A Challenge to Industry in General

I also recommend OSA, sleep deprivation, and sleep disorders awareness training be implemented in all segments of industry. This includes factories, retail outlets, clinics, hospitals, and similar industries where sleep deprivation can cause accidents, injuries, and loss of life. Sleep-related accidents on the highway are not limited to commercial vehicles. Each day automobile drivers have far too many sleep-related accidents while commuting to and from work, while traveling for pleasure, or running errands.

The NCSDR found a profound absence of awareness about sleep disorders and sleep deprivation at every level of society. Physicians, nurses, social workers, teachers, industry leaders, and the general public all need vital information that can lead to the prevention or diagnosis and treatment of sleep problems.

Final Note from Author

When I wrote the first edition of *Snore No More!* in 1990, hardly anything was mentioned on radio, television, or in the newspaper about sleep apnea or other sleep disorders. Little or no attention was devoted to sleep disorder patient awareness.

Sometimes I felt lonely trying to amplify the message toward sleep apnea awareness. Back then, the average person on the street knew little or nothing about sleep apnea. Even today, a large segment of the population is uninformed about sleep apnea and its health hazards.

However, it is now very encouraging to witness some national organizations devoted to patient education by informing the public about sleep apnea and other sleep disorders.

The mission of *Snore No More!* is to heighten the awareness and dangers of sleep apnea, to strongly encourage preventive measures, diagnosis and treatment by board certified sleep specialists.

GLOSSARY

AASM - American Academy of Sleep Medicine.

ABSM - American Board of Sleep Medicine.

AADSM - American Academy of Dental Sleep Medicine, formerly the Academy of Dental Sleep Medicine and previous to Sleep Disorders Dental Society (SDDS).

APAP - Automatic Positive Airway Pressure.

apnea - The stoppage of breath or difficulty in breathing during sleep. A life-threatening sleep disorder. Also called obstructive sleep apnea and OSA in text.

asystole - A condition where the heart stops entirely for as long as six to eight seconds.

Backstopper - An anti-snoring product; a four-inch lightweight ball which is designed to keep the patient off his or her back.

Bilevel - These devices alternate between two different pressures. During inhalation, the pressure is higher in order to keep the airway open. When the patient exhales, a bilevel device drops pressure, making it easier for the patient to exhale.

bradycardia - A slowing of the heart rate.

bronchi - The bronchial tubes.

bruxitis - The act of "grinding" one's teeth while sleeping.

CMD - Craniomandibular Disorders.

central sleep apnea - A less common form of OSA which occurs when the brain fails to send the appropriate signals to the breathing muscles to initiate respiration.

CPAP - Continuous positive airway pressure. A non-invasive anti-snoring device for OSA therapy. Enhances daytime and nighttime breathing by increasing pressure in the airway.

D. ABSM - Diplomate of the American Board of Sleep Medicine

deep sleep stage - The REM, or rapid-eye movement, stage of sleep.

Dental Appliance Therapy - A sequential diagnostic process which matches a patient with an oral appliance designed to improve nighttime breathing by proper positioning of the tongue or jaw. The process involves diagnosis, analysis, and proper fitting by a trained specialist.

deviated septum - A condition in which the partition in the nose is displaced so that it partly blocks one or both nasal passages.

DO - Doctor's degree in osteopathy

EDS - Excessive daytime sleepiness.

endocrinologist - A physician who practices in the field of glandular function.

ENT - An ear, nose, and throat specialist.

expiration - Exhalation.

F.A.C.P. - Fellow of the American College of Physicians

F.C.C.P. - Fellow of the College of Chest Physicians

hypertension - Elevated or high blood pressure.

insomnia - Interruption of sleep or inability to sleep.

inspiration - Inhalation.

laser-assisted uvulopalatoplasty - A surgical procedure used to prevent snoring by using a laser to remove excess tissue from the back of the throat.

LAUP - See laser-assisted uvulopalatoplasty.

Maintenance of Wakefulness Test - A daytime diagnostic test designed to determine whether the sleep disorder involves an abnormal tendency to fall asleep. Also called the **Multiple Sleep Latency Test.**

mandibular - Pertaining to the jaw.

mandibular repositioning device - A device designed to indirectly reposition the tongue by mechanically protruding the jaw.

maxillofacial surgery - Promising surgical advances (not widely available) which enlarge the airway of the soft palate as well as the tongue.

mixed sleep apnea - A combination of Obstructive Sleep Apnea and Central Sleep Apnea.

morbid obesity - The state of weighing more than 20% of one's ideal weight.

M.P.H. - Masters of Public Health.

Multiple Sleep Latency Test - A daytime diagnostic test designed to determine whether the sleep disorder involves an abnormal tendency to fall asleep.

narcolepsy - A congenital or genetic sleep disorder involving a chemical imbalance in the brain cells that control wakefulness and sleep. The patient suffers sudden daytime sleep attacks.

nares - The nostrils.

nasal CPAP - Nasal Continuous Positive Airway Pressure.

nasal polyps - Fleshy growths in the nose.

nasal septum - The thin, flat cartilage and bone that separates the nostrils and nose into its two sides.

NCSDR - The National Commission on Sleep Disorders Research.

NIH - The National Institute of Health.

NHLBI - The National Heart, Lung and Blood Institute.

nocturnal myoclonus - Involuntary muscle twitches, typically very brief occurring repeatedly during sleep, some of which seem to cause arousals from sleep; promoting either difficulty initiating and/or maintaining sleep, and/or excessive daytime sleepiness. (See also **Periodic Limb Movement Disorder**.)

NREM - Non-rapid-eye movement, a stage of sleep.

OA - Oral Appliance.

obstructive sleep apnea - The stoppage of breath or difficulty in breathing during sleep. A life-threatening sleep disorder, OSA occurs when air cannot flow into or out of the sufferer's nose or mouth, although efforts to breathe continue. Also called sleep apnea and OSA in text.

Obstructive sleep hypopnea - Snoring that occurs for 10 seconds or longer which causes a decrease in oxygen in the red blood cells, and typically frequent arousals from sleep.

oropharyngeal tissue - The spot between the base of the tongue and the Adam's apple.

OSA - The stoppage of breath or difficulty in breathing during sleep. A life-threatening sleep disorder. Also called apnea and obstructive sleep apnea in text.

OSAHS – Obstructive Sleep Apnea Hypopnea Syndrome

OSAS - Obstructive Sleep Apnea Syndrome.

OSB - Oral Systemic Balance.

PAP - Positive Airway Pressure.

passive snorer - One who is close to the snorer who suffers from the same fatigue, daytime sleepiness, and other symptoms that the snorer experiences, due to lack of sleep from the snorer's racket.

Periodic Limb Movement Disorder (PLMD) - It is characterized by periodic episodes of repetitive and highly stereotyped limb movements that occur during sleep. The muscle twitches last .5 to 5.0 seconds. (See also nocturnal myclonus and Restless Legs Syndrome.)

polysomnogram - A medical test which measures physiological functions during sleep. Used to determine whether sleep disorders are present in the snorer.

REM - The rapid-eye movement stage of sleep.

REM behavior disorder - A condition involving abnormal, often violent, movements during sleep.

Restless Legs Syndrome (RLS) - Recurring, uncomfortable to painful feelings in the legs that result in uncontrollable urges to move the legs when awake (especially when sitting, lying down or standing in one place). Exercise and stretching the leg muscles helps to relieve some of this discomfort. At night, the patient typically has Periodic Limb Movement Disorder. (See also Periodic Limb Movement Disorder.)

rhinitis - Inflammation of the mucus membranes of the nasal passage.

R.Psg.T. - Registered Polysomnography Technologist, trained and certified in all technical aspects of sleep evaluations by the Association of Polysomnographic Technologists.

SCOR - Specialized Center of Research, a project on breathing disorders of sleep funded by the NIH.

SIDS - Sudden Infant Death Syndrome, death in infants due to the stoppage of breath.

sinusitis - Inflammation of the sinuses.

sleep disorders center - A diagnostic and/or treatment facility staffed by sleep disorders medicine specialists and technicians.

snorer's disease - A non-technical term used to describe the snoring disorder.

snoring - The sound made by air passing through irregularities and narrowings in the throat and windpipe. Loud, erratic snoring can be indicative of the presence of a serious disorder, sleep apnea.

SNOR.X - An anti-snoring Tongue Retaining Device (TRD) that helps reduce loud snoring in non-apneic patients.

soft palate - The posterior, or back, part of the palate.

TMD Temporomandibular Disorders (or dysfunction).

TMJ - Temporomandibular joint, the area of connection between the temporal and mandibular bones.

trachea - The windpipe.

tracheostomy - A surgical procedure used only in patients with severe, life-threatening OSA. It involves opening and inserting an air tube into the trachea.

TRD - Tongue retaining device; used to position the tongue in such a way as to aid in clearing the airway for more efficient breathing.

Upper Airway Resistance Syndrome (UARS) - Apparent obstructed breathing without a decrease in arterial oxygen as measured by a pulse oximeter associated with frequent arousals from sleep.

UPPP - See uvulopalatopharyngeoplasty.

uvula - Small, soft tissue that hangs from the soft palate.

uvulopalatopharyngeoplasty - A surgical procedure used to stop snoring by removing excess tissue at the back of the throat.

VA - Veterans Administration or Veterans Affairs

REFERENCES

Breathing Disorders During Sleep, a brochure published by the National Heart, Lung and Blood Institute, National Institute of Health.

The Effects of a Nonsurgical Treatment for Obstructive Sleep Apnea, the Tongue Retaining Device, Rosalind D. Cartwright, Ph.D., Charles F. Samuelson, M.D., JAMA, August 13, 1982: Vol. 248, No. 6.

The Efficacy of Surgical Modifications of the Upper Airway in Adults with Obstructive Sleep Apnea Syndrome, Aaron E. Sher, Kenneth B. Schechtman and Jay F. Piccirillo, November 1995.

Facts About Sleep Apnea: National Heart, Lung and Blood Institute, March 2005.

From Obstructive Sleep Apnea Syndrome to Upper Airway Resistance Syndrome: Consistency of Daytime Sleepiness, Christian Guilleminasult, Riccardo Stoohs, Alex Clerk, Jerald Simons and Michael Labanowski. July 1992.

Health Insurance Carriers, VA & You, the Nonservice-Connected Veteran, Department of Veterans Affairs.

Helping You Choose Quality Ambulatory Care and How You Choose Quality Hospital Care, Joint Commission on Accreditation of Healthcare Organizations.

Oral Appliance Therapy for Snoring and Obstructive Sleep Apnea: Academy of Dental Sleep Medicine, 2004.

Oral Appliances for the Treatment of Snoring and Obstructive Sleep Apnea: A Review and *Practice Parameters for the Treatment of Snoring and Obstructive Sleep Apnea With Oral Appliances,* 2007, American Academy of Sleep Medicine.

Practice Parameters for the Use of Laser-Assisted Uvulopalatoplasty, an American Sleep Disorders Association report, August 1994.

Public Health Service Assessment—Continuous Positive Airway pressure for the Treatment of Obstructive Sleep Apnea in Adults, Prepared by OSHA/NCHSR/OHTA/HHANDELSMAN/4/23/87.

Recognition of Obstructive Sleep Apnea, Kingman P. Strohl and Susan Redline, November 9, 1995 and revised from February 5, 1996.

SIDS—"Back to Sleep" Campaign—NIH, National Institute of Child Health & Human Development - Revised November 2005.

Significance and Treatment of Nonapneic Snoring, Patrick J. Strollo, Jr. and Mark H. Sanders.

Sleep Apnea: Is Your Patient at Risk?, National Institutes of Health—National Heart, Lung and Blood Institute. *Reprint September 1999.*

Sleep Apnea, Sleepiness and Driving Risk, The American Thoracic Society — Medical section of the American Lung Association. This official statement of the American Thoracic Society (ATS) was adopted by the ATS Board of Directors, June 1994.

Sleep Thief, Restless Legs Syndrome, Virginia N. Wilson (ED: A.S. Walters, M.D.), 1996

Sleep Thieves, Stanley Coren.

Snoring: A Medical Perspective, Causes and Treatments, Meir Kryger, M.D., Martin Scharf, Ph.D., Daniel E. Cohen, M.D., Kingman Strohl, M.D.

State of the Art—Physiologic Basis of Therapy for Sleep Apnea, Kingman P. Strohl, Neil S. Cherniack and Barbara Gothe: AM REM RESPIR DIS 1968: 134:791-802.

The Dental/Medical Connection—Snoring and Sleep Apnea: Facts about oral airway appliances. TmData Resources, 2005.

Upper Airway Resistance Syndrome. Sick, Symptomatic but Under Recognized, Ralph Downey III, Ronald M. Perkin and Joanne MacQuarrie. June 1993.

Wake Up America: A National Sleep Alert—A report of the National Commission on Sleep Disorders Research, submitted to the United States Congress and the Secretary, U.S. Department of Health and Human Services, Volume One and Two.

What is Sleep Apnea?—The American Sleep Apnea Association.

You and Your Stuffy Nose, American Academy of Otolaryngology—Head and Neck Surgery, Inc., 1985.

PROFESSIONAL CONTRIBUTORS

R. Michael Alvarez, DDS, has a private practice in Fremont, California. Presenter of seminars and training on the collaboration of medical and dental professionals in the delivery of oral appliances for treating sleep disorders. Certified provider of the Oral Systemic Balance Therapy and board certified by the American Academy of Dental Sleep Medicine (AADSM). A founding member and past president of the AADSM and cofounder of the Medical and Dental Educational Network. Inventor of the Snorex, an anti-snoring tongue-retaining device.

Lawrence E. Kline, DO, FACP, FCCP, D. ABSM, is the Director and Senior Consultant at Scripps Clinic Sleep Center, Division of Chest and Critical Care Medicine, La Jolla, California.

Robert R. Rogers, DMD, is the Director of Dental Medicine for St. Barnabas Medical Center in Gibsonia, Pennsylvania. He has had a special interest in the treatment of sleep disordered breathing since 1990 and treats patients in conjunction with many regional sleep centers.

Dr. Rogers is the founding president of the American Academy of Dental Sleep Medicine (AADSM) and served again as president in 1995 and 1999. In addition to being a member of the Board of Directors over 10 years, he chaired the Education and Curriculum Committee for 6 years and was the director of the AADSM Resource Center 12 years. Dr. Rogers is a diplomate of the American Board of Dental Sleep Medicine and is the recipient of the AADSM Distinguished Service Award.

Dr. Rogers is the author/editor of the AADSM educational slide series and is a contributing author to the graduate dental text, *Clark's Clinical Dentistry.* He is currently the dental consultant to Respironics, Inc. Most recently, Dr. Rogers was a member of the task force for the revision of the AASM Position Paper and Practice Parameters on Oral Appliance Therapy.

Arthur M. Strauss, DDS, Doctor of Integrative Medicine, Healer, Founding Member and Past President of Sleep Disorders Dental Society (SDDS), now known as the American Academy of Dental Sleep Medicine (AADSM); Chairperson, AADSM Professional Relations Committee. Author of "Oral Devices for the Management of Snoring and Obstructive Sleep Apnea" from the text, *Snoring and Obstructive Sleep Apnea,* Second Edition, David N.F. Fairbanks, MD.

Kingman P. Strohl, MD, D. ABSM is the Director of the Center for Sleep Disorders Research, Case Western Reserve University and University Hospital of Cleveland, Ohio. Director of a Specialized Center of Research project on breathing disorders of sleep. He was the 1996 President of The American Sleep Apnea Association. He has authored or coauthored over 100 publications on a variety of subjects regarding OSA, sleepiness and driving risk, and the control of breathing in children and adults.

Contact Information for Patients and Doctors

Patients who want to locate a licensed OSB dentist or want more information on OSB Therapy should call the toll free number listed below.

Doctors can become certified as OSB practitioners after a series of courses and upon meeting specific educational and practical requirements. Those interested in receiving OSB training may call the toll free number listed below for additional information.

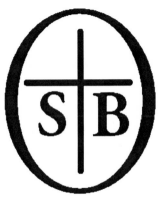

Oral Systemic Balance®
Therapeutic Systems

Oral Systemic Balance®
1901 South Union Avenue, Suite B5010
Tacoma, Washington 98405
www.oralsystemicbalance.com
Phone: (800) 977-1945
Fax: (253) 272-0489

SPONSORSHIP

I want to extend my sincere thanks to the Respironics Sleep and
Respiratory Research Foundation for their generous
participation in sponsoring the Fourth edition of *Snore No More!*

I salute the Foundation in its involvement in the advancement of
sleep disorders awareness, research and respiratory health.

James L. Mosley – author/publisher

The Respironics Sleep and Respiratory Research Foundation

The Respironics Sleep and Respiratory Research
Foundation awards funds for charitable, scientific,
literary and educational opportunities that promote
awareness of, and research into, the medical
consequences of sleep and respiratory problems.
Established in 2003, the Foundation is a qualified
Section 501(c)(3) not-for-profit organization that
provides grants for sleep and respiratory
research. The Respironics Sleep and Respiratory
Research Foundation is a private foundation that
is sponsored by Respironics, Inc.

Printed in the United States
127383LV00001B/24/A

9 781884 687679